Cosmetic and Clinical Applications of Botox® and Dermal Fillers

Second Edition

William J. Lipham, MD, FACS

Ophthalmic Plastic and Reconstructive Surgeon
Minnesota Eye Consultants, PA
Minneapolis, Minnesota
Adjunct Associate Professor
Division of Ophthalmic Plastic and Reconstructive Surgery
Department of Ophthalmology
University of Minnesota School of Medicine
Minneapolis, Minnesota

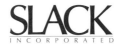

SLACK
INCORPORATED

*Delivering the best in health care information
and education worldwide*

www.slackbooks.com

ISBN: 978-1-55642-796-1

Cover illustration by Lauren Shavell of Medical Imagery.

The procedures and practices described in this book should be implemented in a manner consistent with the professional standards set for the circumstances that apply in each specific situation. Every effort has been made to confirm the accuracy of the information presented and to correctly relate generally accepted practices. The authors, editor, and publisher cannot accept responsibility for errors or exclusions or for the outcome of the material presented herein. There is no expressed or implied warranty of this book or information imparted by it. Care has been taken to ensure that drug selection and dosages are in accordance with currently accepted/recommended practice. Due to continuing research, changes in government policy and regulations, and various effects of drug reactions and interactions, it is recommended that the reader carefully review all materials and literature provided for each drug, especially those that are new or not frequently used. Any review or mention of specific companies or products is not intended as an endorsement by the author or publisher.

SLACK Incorporated uses a review process to evaluate submitted material. Prior to publication, educators or clinicians provide important feedback on the content that we publish. We welcome feedback on this work.

Contact SLACK Incorporated for more information about other books in this field or about the availability of our books from distributors outside the United States.

Published by: SLACK Incorporated
                  6900 Grove Road
                  Thorofare, NJ 08086 USA
                  Telephone: 856-848-1000
                  Fax: 856-853-5991
                  www.slackbooks.com

Library of Congress Cataloging-in-Publication Data

Lipham, William J., 1964-
  Cosmetic and clinical applications of botox and dermal fillers / William J. Lipham. -- 2nd ed.
      p. ; cm.
  Rev. ed. of: Cosmetic and clinical applications of botulinum toxin. 2004.
  Includes bibliographical references and index.
    ISBN 978-1-55642-796-1 (alk. paper)
    1. Botulinum toxin--Therapeutic use. 2. Skin--Wrinkles--Chemotherapy. I. Lipham, William J., 1964- Cosmetic and clinical applications of botulinum toxin. II. Title.
    [DNLM: 1. Botulinum Toxins--therapeutic use. 2. Cosmetic Techniques. 3. Facial Muscles--drug effects. QW 630.5.B2 L764c 2007]

  RL120.B66L55 2007
  615'.778--dc22
                              2007026513

Printed in the United States of America.

Last digit is print number: 10 9 8 7 6 5 4 3 2 1

Dedication

To my mother, for her support and encouragement to pursue my chosen career in medicine, and my father, who was an outstanding teacher, author, and role model. I would also like to thank my wife, Azura, and my daughter, Chloe, for their patience and understanding while I toiled away on this book, as well as for the joy and happiness that they bring to me each and every day!

Contents

Acknowledgments

After a lot of hard work on a project like this, one of the best parts is having the opportunity to pause, reflect, and recognize the individuals and events that have had a positive impact on your personal and professional life. I have been very fortunate to have had the opportunity to work with and train under some truly remarkable individuals. I would, therefore, like to thank my two most significant academic mentors and role models: Dr. Igal Gery, who taught me to enjoy life every day and to seek my goals one small step at a time, and Dr. Jonathan J. Dutton, who expertly taught me the art and science of oculoplastic surgery that I strive to pass on to a future generation of residents in training.

In addition, I would like to thank my colleagues at work (the troops in the trenches) who have contributed very significantly to the production of this text—among them are my administrative assistant, Renee Adkins, and my nursing and technical support staff at Minnesota Eye Consultants. Their positive attitude and hard work ethic make my job a pleasure.

About the Author

William J. Lipham, MD, FACS is an ophthalmic plastic and reconstructive surgeon who performs reconstructive surgery on the eyelids, tear drainage system, and orbit. In addition to managing complex medical and surgical cases, he also provides a broad array of facial rejuvenation services, including cosmetic eyelid surgery, laser skin resurfacing, and small incision endoscopic forehead lifts, as well as botulinum toxin and dermal filler injections for wrinkle reduction.

Dr. Lipham received his medical degree from Baylor College of Medicine in Houston, Tex and performed his transitional internship at the University of Hawaii, Honolulu, Hawaii where he met his wife, Azura. He then completed a 3-year ophthalmology residency at the Bascom Palmer Eye Institute of the University of Miami, Fla and went on to perform an additional 2-year American Society of Ophthalmic Plastic and Reconstructive Surgery (ASOPRS) fellowship with Jonathan J. Dutton, MD, PhD at Duke University Eye Center in Durham, NC. Upon completion of his fellowship, Dr. Lipham was selected by the residents and faculty of Duke University Eye Center to receive the Hornaday Fellow Award for demonstrating excellence in clinical care, resident education, ethics, and research. He was also the recipient of the Marvin H. Quickert Award, which is given for the most outstanding thesis from those submitted by candidates seeking membership in the ASOPRS.

Dr. Lipham is a Fellow of the American Board of Ophthalmology and American College of Surgeons (FACS). He is an active member of the ASOPRS, the American Academy of Ophthalmology, and the American Medical Association. He currently is the secretary of the Minnesota Academy of Ophthalmology and is a past president of the Minneapolis Ophthalmological Society. In addition to these activities, he is a surgical consultant for a number of medical device companies, is a frequent lecturer at scientific meetings, and has published numerous articles and chapters in the fields of ophthalmology and oculoplastic surgery.

Contributing Authors

Gregg S. Gayre, MD
Chief, Division of Ophthalmic Plastic and Reconstructive Surgery
Department of Ophthalmology
Kaiser Permanente Medical Center
San Rafael, Calif

David B. Granet, MD
Associate Professor
Ann Ratner Chair, Division of Pediatric Ophthalmology and Adult Strabismus
Department of Ophthalmology
University of California—San Diego School of Medicine
La Jolla, Calif

Patrick K. Johnson, MD
Ophthalmology Resident
University of Minnesota
Twin Cities, Minn

David R. Jordan, MD
Professor
Chief, Division of Ophthalmic Plastic and Reconstructive Surgery
Department of Ophthalmology
University of Ottawa School of Medicine
Ottawa, Ontario, Canada

Don O. Kikkawa, MD
Professor
Chief, Division of Ophthalmic Facial Plastic Surgery
Department of Ophthalmology
University of California—San Diego School of Medicine
La Jolla, Calif

Michael S. McCracken, MD
Clinical Instructor
Division of Ophthalmic Facial Plastic Surgery
Department of Ophthalmology
University of California—San Diego School of Medicine
La Jolla, Calif

Preface

While botulinum toxin has been safely and effectively used for the treatment of a variety of functional medical disorders since the 1980s, there has been a recent explosion of interest with respect to its cosmetic applications. This interest has stemmed in large part from the recent Food and Drug Administration approval of BOTOX® (Allergan Inc, Irvine, Calif) in the United States for the treatment of glabellar furrows or "frown lines." It should be noted, however, that physicians have been and are actively performing a wide variety of additional cosmetic treatments with botulinum toxin albeit in an "off-label" fashion. These additional areas commonly include transverse forehead lines, orbicularis rhytides or "crow's feet," perioral or "smoker's" lines, and melomental or "marionette" lines.

Since botulinum toxin exerts its effect by inactivating muscle contraction, its cosmetic indications have been directed toward reducing lines of active facial expression. These lines or wrinkles slowly develop over a number of years during which an individual has performed thousands of repetitive facial expressions. As such, botulinum toxin injections are generally felt to serve as a form of preventive maintenance for lines that develop due to repetitive muscular contraction. Therefore, the age demographic for individuals pursuing cosmetic botulinum toxin injections is typically younger than those seeking surgical intervention for other cosmetic indications since they are trying to prevent the lines from forming in the first place.

In addition to the broad array of cosmetic applications for botulinum toxin, a new range of functional treatments is similarly beginning to emerge. These treatments include creating a "chemical" tarsorrhaphy to promote corneal healing, reducing thyroid-associated eyelid retraction, and, most compelling, reducing the frequency and severity of muscle tension and migraine headaches. These new applications significantly expand the scope of botulinum toxin treatments for medical disorders that have traditionally included the treatment of strabismus as well as a number of disorders of spasticity.

The text also describes how to perform a broad range of treatments with a wide variety of dermal filler agents, including the newer hyaluronic acid and poly-l-lactic acid derivatives. This new generation of dermal fillers is very exciting because it provides excellent results with reduced potential for inducing an allergic reaction. It should be noted that unlike botulinum toxin injections, which are used to treat lines of active facial expression, dermal filler agents are typically used to treat lines that are present at rest or to fill areas such as the lip line and depressed scars.

It is the intent and purpose of the authors of this text to familiarize readers with botulinum toxin treatments and dermal filler agents and provide useful guidelines and helpful advice with regard to their clinical implementation. This should not, however, serve as a substitute for personal instruction and training, which is absolutely necessary before physicians can begin to pursue or offer treatments to their patients. It is the authors' intention that this text should be used to supplement the reader's training and serve as a readily accessible clinical reference that can be used to concisely review the subject material.

Textbooks provide facts and details organized in a systematic and step-by-step fashion; however, it is difficult to learn the actual techniques without seeing it performed. The accompanying DVD complements the textbook content with narrated video examples of certain techniques. The DVD format was used in order to showcase higher resolution video along with the ability to select and assess particular chapters in any order. We have combined the DVD with the more thorough explanations in this textbook in order to overcome the limitations of learning from a single instructional format alone.

It should also be noted that none of the companies that commercially produce botulinum toxin or dermal filler agents have provided financial support for this text and, therefore, it does not reflect their policies or opinions on this subject matter.

William J. Lipham, MD, FACS

CHAPTER 1

A Brief History of the Clinical Applications of Botulinum Toxin

William J. Lipham, MD, FACS

Like most advances in medical therapy, the cosmetic and clinical applications of botulinum toxin type-A are the result of numerous individuals who observed clinical conditions and were able to translate these findings into significant medical advances. The organism *Clostridium botulinum* was originally isolated by Professor E. Van Ermengem in 1895 after members of a music club in Elezelles, Belgium sustained systemic paralysis following the consumption of rare-cooked, salted ham, leading to the death of 3 members of their group.[1] In the 20 years that followed the initial discovery of *Clostridium botulinum*, different strains of the organism were identified that were felt to produce distinct forms of botulinum toxin.[2] Initial attempts to purify the causative agent from the organism that induced muscular paralysis were unsuccessful. Dr. Herman Sommer of the Hooper Foundation, University of California was unable to produce a purified form of botulinum toxin but was the first investigator to extract a sludge-like precipitate that was capable of inducing paralysis in laboratory animals. In 1946, Dr. Edward Schantz and his associates at Camp Detrick, Md succeeded in purifying botulinum toxin type-A toxin in crystallized form.[3] This led to subsequent investigations into the mechanism of action of botulinum toxin type-A, which was first described by Dr. Vernon Brooks who established that muscle paralysis was due to a blockade of the release of acetylcholine (ACh) from the motor endplate at the myoneural junction.

Clinical Applications

The first investigator to pursue the clinical application of botulinum toxin was Dr. Alan Scott of the Smith-Kettlewell Eye Research Foundation in San Francisco, Calif. In the late 1960s and early 1970s, Dr. Scott attempted to weaken the extraocular muscles of monkeys with botulinum toxin type-A and other chemical agents with the hope that these compounds could eventually be used for the nonsurgical treatment of strabismus in humans. His interest in finding compounds for this study led him to correspond with Dr. Schantz, who provided Dr. Scott with botulinum toxin type-A for his initial and subsequent investigations into this area.[4] The results of his first primate studies, which were published in 1973, confirmed that botulinum toxin type-A was the most effective of the agents that he had investigated to weaken extraocular muscles.[5] In the discussion section of the same paper, Dr. Scott postulated that botulinum toxin type-A might also be useful for the nonsurgical correction of a wide variety of musculoskeletal disorders as well as a potential treatment for muscle spasticity. It is worth noting that these initial predictions were made before botulinum toxin had ever been injected into humans for experimental or clinical purposes.

Dr. Scott was also the first individual to demonstrate the clinical effectiveness of botulinum toxin type-A for the treatment of strabismus in humans in a landmark paper published in 1980.[6] During this period, Dr. Scott also founded a company named Oculinum, Inc to develop and test botulinum toxin type-A. In addition to the nonsurgical treatment of strabismus, botulinum toxin was subsequently approved for the treatment of numerous disorders of spasticity, including blepharospasm, hemifacial spasm, and Meige syndrome, in December 1989. Clinical indications for use were subsequently expanded to also include the treatment of cervical dystonia and spasmodic torticollis. After purchasing Oculinum, Inc in 1991, Allergan Inc (Irvine, Calif) renamed botulinum toxin type-A simply as BOTOX®. The clinical effectiveness of botulinum toxin eventually led to the worldwide approval of BOTOX for the previously mentioned indications.

In 1991, a different preparation of botulinum toxin type-A named Dysport® (Ipsen Limited, Britain) was approved for the treatment of cervical dystonia and movement disorders in Europe and Asia, but it is currently unavailable in the United States and Canada. More recently, in 2001, botulinum toxin type-B, MYOBLOC® (Solstice Neurosciences, Inc, San Francisco, Calif) was Food and Drug Administration (FDA)–approved for use in the United States for the treatment of cervical dystonia.

Cosmetic Applications

The first scientific abstract and publication discussing the cosmetic applications of botulinum toxin was published by Alastair and Jean Carruthers in 1992[7]; however, these authors note that their initial investigations into the cosmetic applications of botulinum toxin were based on discussions they had in the mid 1980s with Dr. Scott who reported to them that he had treated a patient with botulinum toxin to reduce the appearance of facial lines. Dr. Jean Carruthers had similarly observed that patients that she had treated for blepharospasm demonstrated a reduction in the appearance of their glabellar furrows, which was attributed to chemical inactivation of the brow depressor muscles. Based on her observations, the Carruthers achieved their first encouraging cosmetic results by administering a single injection of botulinum toxin type-A into their secretary's forehead. Their subsequent clinical trial found that 16 of 17 patients showed clinical reduction of their glabellar lines for periods of 3 to 11 months.

At approximately the same time, a group at Columbia University described that they had observed a reduction in the appearance of dynamic lines of facial expression in individuals who had undergone BOTOX treatments for facial dystonia.[8] They also performed the first double-blind, placebo-controlled study for the treatment for hyperkinetic facial lines.[9] Subsequently, a number of authors started to investigate the potential cosmetic applications of botulinum toxin to include treatment of "crow's feet," transverse forehead lines, and platysmal bands.[10,11] Since that time, more subtle modifications have been described for the treatment of perioral lines and the correction of hyperhidrosis.[12-14] None of the treatments were initially FDA–approved and were considered an off-label indication for the use of botulinum toxin; however, on April 15, 2002, BOTOX received FDA approval for the nonsurgical reduction of glabellar furrows, or "frown" lines, based on a large, double-blind, randomized study of 553 patients recruited in a multicenter trial.[15] In the past 5 to 7 years, there has been an explosion of interest in this area by the public as well as physicians. The initial public reaction was guarded toward the cosmetic use of BOTOX. Today, BOTOX is now commonly described in the lay press and actively pursued by millions of individuals within the United States and around the world.[16]

References

1. Klein AW. Botulinum toxins: introduction. *Semin Cutan Med Surg.* 2001;20(2):69-70.
2. Carruthers A. Botulinum toxin type-A: history and current cosmetic use in the upper face. *Dis Mon.* 2002;48(5):299-322.
3. Klein AW. Cosmetic therapy with botulinum toxin: anecdotal memoirs. *Dermatol Surg.* 1996;22(9):757-759.
4. Carruthers A, Carruthers J. Botulinum toxin type-A: history and current cosmetic use in the upper face. *Semin Cutan Med Surg.* 2001;20(2):71-84.
5. Scott AB, Rosenbaum AL, Collins CC. Pharmacologic weakening of extraocular muscles. *Invest Ophthalmol Vis Sci.* 1973;12:924-927.
6. Scott AB. Botulinum toxin injection into extraocular muscles as an alternative to strabismus surgery. *Ophthalmology.* 1980;87:1044-1049.
7. Carruthers JD, Carruthers JA. Treatment of glabellar frown lines with *C. botulinum*-A exotoxin. *J Dermatol Surg Oncol.* 1992;18(1):17-21.
8. Blitzer A, Brin MF, Keen MS, Aviv JE. Botulinum toxin for the treatment of hyperfunctional lines of the face. *Arch Otolaryngol Head Neck Surg.* 1993;119(9):1018-1022.
9. Keen M, Blitzer A, Aviv J, et al. Botulinum toxin type-A for hyperkinetic facial lines: results of a double-blind, placebo-controlled study. *Plast Reconstr Surg.* 1994;94(1):94-99.
10. Kane MA. Nonsurgical treatment of platysmal bands with injection of botulinum toxin type-A. *Plast Reconstr Surg.* 1999;103(2):656-663, discussion 664-655.
11. Klein AW. Treatment of wrinkles with Botox. *Curr Probl Dermatol.* 2002;30:188-217.
12. Brandt FS, Bellman B. Cosmetic use of botulinum A exotoxin for the aging neck. *Dermatol Surg.* 1998;24(11):1232-1234.
13. Fagien S, Brandt FS. Primary and adjunctive use of botulinum toxin type A (Botox) in facial aesthetic surgery: beyond the glabella. *Clin Plast Surg.* 2001;28(1):127-148.
14. Odderson IR. Hyperhidrosis treated by botulinum A exotoxin. *Dermatol Surg.* 1998;24:1237-1241.
15. Carruthers JA, Lowe NJ, Menter MA, et al. A multicenter, double-blind, randomized, placebo-controlled study of the efficacy and safety of botulinum toxin type A in the treatment of glabellar lines. *J Am Acad Dermatol.* 2002;46(6):840-849.
16. Noonan D, Adler J. The botox boom. *Newsweek.* 2002;139(19):50-56, 58.

CHAPTER 2

What Is Botulinum Toxin and How Does It Work?

William J. Lipham, MD, FACS

Physical Properties

There are 7 distinct strains of *Clostridium botulinum* that have been identified. Each strain is characterized by the type of botulinum neurotoxin that it is capable of producing and has been classified as type A, B, C, D, E, F, or G.[1] While all of these neurotoxins inhibit the release of ACh at the myoneural junction, they all vary in their chemical structure and size as well as their mechanism of action within the nerve terminal itself. Five of these subtypes (A, B, E, F, G) affect the human nervous system, while 2 subtypes (C and D) do not. Types A and B are the 2 most clinically relevant subtypes and, therefore, are commercially produced. Botulinum toxin type-A is felt to exert the most powerful neuromuscular blockade and is also capable of exerting its effect for the longest duration of time.[2] In contrast, botulinum toxin type-E and type-F are also capable of blocking myoneural transmission, but they have a shorter duration of action when compared to types A and B and, therefore, are not commercially produced.

Both botulinum toxin type-A and type-B are composed of a 150 kD polypeptide consisting of a disulfide bond-linked light chain and heavy chain.[3] These disulfide-linked molecules are associated with other non-neurotoxin proteins during their synthesis to form a neurotoxin complex, which is approximately 500 kD in size (Figure 2-1). These non-neurotoxin accessory proteins may serve a beneficial role in stabilizing the fragile botulinum toxin molecule when it is reconstituted.

Mechanism of Action

At the neuromuscular junction, the motor nerve terminal lies in close apposition with the adjacent muscle fiber. When botulinum toxin is administered, the heavy chain binds selectively to cell membrane receptors on the outer surface of the presynaptic nerve terminal (Figure 2-2). The entire neurotoxin complex (both light and heavy chains) is then internalized into the nerve terminal via receptor-mediated endocytosis (Figure 2-3). The vesicles containing the botulinum toxin then fuse with digestive vacuoles that cleave the botulinum toxin molecule into separate light and heavy chains.[4,5]

Figure 2-1. The botulinum toxin molecule consists of a light chain and heavy chain joined by a single disulfide bond. While the heavy chain is responsible for binding to the nerve terminal receptors, the light chain exerts its effect by preventing the release of ACh from the nerve terminal.

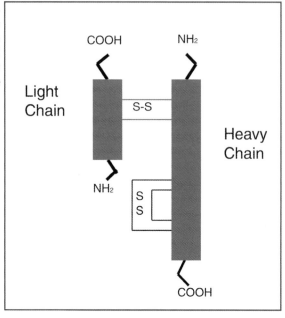

Figure 2-2. The heavy chain of the botulinum toxin molecule binds selectively to cell membrane receptors on the outer surface of the nerve terminal. (Used by permission © 2003 Allergan, Inc.)

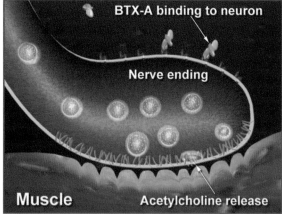

Figure 2-3. The entire neurotoxin complex is then internalized into the motor nerve terminal through receptor-mediated endocytosis. (Used by permission © 2003 Allergan, Inc.)

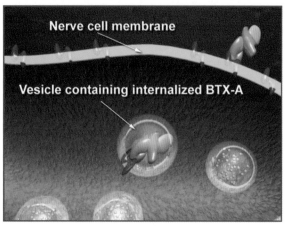

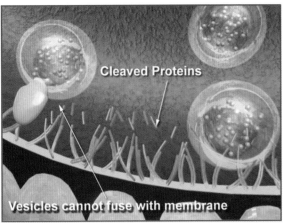

Cleaved Proteins

Vesicles cannot fuse with membrane

Figure 2-4. The light chain exerts its effect by cleaving the synaptic neural-associated protein (SNAP-25) that is responsible for fusion of vesicles containing ACh with the nerve terminal cell membrane. (Used by permission © 2003 Allergan, Inc.)

The light chain exerts the paralytic effect of botulinum toxin by inactivating a group of proteins that are responsible for the fusion of vesicles containing the neurotransmitter ACh with the nerve cell membrane and thereby blocking the release of ACh into the neuromuscular junction. This group of proteins is referred to as the SNARE complex (soluble N-ethylmalemide-sensitive factor attachment protein receptor), a neural exocytic complex that regulates the membrane docking and fusion of synaptic vesicles and the release of ACh.[6]

Each botulinum toxin serotype acts upon the SNARE complex. Serotypes A, C, and E cleave the synaptic neural-associated protein (SNAP-25) molecule, while serotypes B, D, F, and G cleave synaptobrevin or vesicle-associated membrane protein (VAMP), each at a distinct site (Figure 2-4). In each case, botulinum toxin enzymatically inactivates a specific protein that is required for the docking and fusion of vesicles containing ACh into the neuromuscular junction.[7] The inhibition of ACh release results in localized muscle weakness (paralysis) that gradually reverses over time. The mechanism by which botulinum toxin-induced muscle weakness is reversed is unknown, but it may involve the intraneural turnover of the affected docking proteins (responsible for the release of ACh into the neuromuscular junction), the sprouting of new nerve terminals, or a combination of both of these mechanisms.[8]

The axon begins to expand approximately 2 months after administration of botulinum toxin, and new nerve terminal sprouts emerge and extend toward the muscle surface.[9] The motor nerve unit is re-established once a new sprout forms a physical synaptic connection with the previous neuromuscular junction. The new nerve sprouts that do not establish a connection to the motor endplate, however, subsequently regress and are spontaneously eliminated while the parent, or former, nerve terminal is re-established (Figure 2-5).[10]

An understanding of the mechanism of action of botulinum toxin allows one to understand the time required for the onset of paralysis as well as the duration of clinical effect. Botulinum toxin, once injected, takes approximately 3 to 4 days for its effect to become clinically apparent. This corresponds to the amount of time that is required for the botulinum toxin molecule to bind to the motor nerve terminal, undergo internalization via receptor-mediated endocytosis, and block ACh release through inactivation of the SNAP-25 or VAMP proteins.

In contrast, the clinical duration of effect, which is approximately 3 to 4 months in length, corresponds to the time that is required for new sprouts to grow from the nerve root to re-establish the motor endplate. Therefore, the duration of effect is not dependent

Figure 2-5. Approximately 2 months after injection, the nerve terminal begins to expand and new sprouts emerge and extend toward the muscle surface. Additional redundant nerve sprouts are also produced. The motor nerve unit is re-established once a new sprout forms a physical synaptic connection with the previous neuromuscular junction. (Used by permission © 2003 Allergan, Inc.)

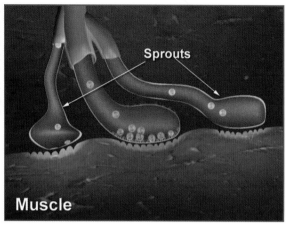

on the continued presence of botulinum toxin at the nerve terminal, but rather reflects the length of time that it takes for a particular individual's nerves to regenerate and develop a functional connection at the myoneural junction.[11]

Contraindications and Precautions

The only contraindication to the administration of botulinum toxin includes neuromuscular disease such as myasthenia gravis or Eaton-Lambert syndrome, which can similarly potentiate the effects of botulinum toxin.[12] Similarly, botulinum toxin should not be administered to individuals with a cutaneous infection at the proposed site of injection. Since the effects of botulinum toxin on pregnancy in human subjects are unknown, administration during pregnancy or while breast feeding is not recommended. Similarly, botulinum toxin is not recommended for use in children. Finally, both compounds contain human albumin to stabilize the lyopholite; therefore, individuals with allergies to eggs should not receive botulinum toxin because there may be an increased risk for an anaphylactic reaction to the albumin proteins. Epinephrine should always be available if an anaphylactic reaction should occur.

Clinicians should obtain a complete list of current medications from patients undergoing botulinum toxin injections. Drug interactions can occur with botulinum toxin, and special care or postponement of treatment should be considered in patients taking aminoglycosides, which can potentiate the effect of botulinum toxin and produce a botulism-like clinical syndrome. In contrast, aminoquinolines may delay the onset of botulinum toxin.

Adverse Reactions

The most common adverse events in clinical trials of BOTOX included headache, respiratory infection, flu syndrome, blepharoptosis, and nausea.[13] While weakness of the injected muscle is expected following botulinum toxin administration, inadvertent administration of larger doses to the effected area may induce severe paresis or paralysis of the muscle, which may cause problems for the patient. For example, when botulinum toxin is administered to the periocular region for the treatment of blepharospasm, the rate and strength of the blink response may be compromised or lagophthalmos may develop due to weakness of the orbicularis oculi muscle. This may result in corneal exposure, ad ocular irritation, and redness, which should be treated with aggressive lubrication of the ocular surface. Similarly, weakening of the orbicularis oris muscle may compromise an individual's ability to purse his or her lips or maintain a symmetric smile.

Botulinum toxin may also inadvertently spread to involve adjacent muscles with a variety of untoward side effects. A thorough understanding of facial muscle anatomy and proper injection technique is the best way to avoid these problems. Transient upper eyelid ptosis is probably the most common example of this type of adverse event and may develop following inactivation of the orbicularis oculi muscle in blepharospasm or hemifacial spasm patients. The ptosis results from diffusion or inadvertent administration of botulinum toxin behind the orbital septum, which weakens the levator palpebrae superioris muscle. Less commonly, injection into the platysmal bands in the neck region may temporarily induce dysphonia or dysphagia.

If eyelid ptosis occurs, a single drop of apraclonidine 0.5% may be administered 3 times daily to temporarily stimulate Müller's muscle, which elevates the eyelid, until the ptosis resolves. Similarly, over-the-counter preparations containing the vasoconstrictor naphazoline (eg, Naphcon-A® [Alcon Canada, Mississauga, Ontario], naphazoline hydrochloride) may demonstrate a beneficial effect. Patients should be warned, however, about the possibility of rebound vasodilation when vasoconstrictors are discontinued, resulting in slightly inflamed eyes.

References

1. Jankovic J. Botulinum A toxin in the treatment of blepharospasm. *Adv Neurol.* 1988;49:467-472.
2. Hankins CL, Strimling R, Rogers GS. Botulinum A toxin for glabellar wrinkles: dose and response. *Dermatol Surg.* 1998;24(11):1181-1183.
3. Lew MF. Review of the FDA-approved uses of botulinum toxins, including data suggesting efficacy in pain reduction. *Clin J Pain.* 2002;18(6 Suppl):S142-S146.
4. Pearce LB, First ER, MacCallum RD, Gupta A. Pharmacologic characterization of botulinum toxin for basic science and medicine. *Toxicon.* 1997;35(9):1373-1412.
5. Lowe NJ, Yamauchi PS, Lask GP, Patnaik R, Moore D. Botulinum toxins types A and B for brow furrows: preliminary experiences with type B toxin dosing. *J Cosmet Laser Ther.* 2002;4(1):15-18.
6. Setler P. The biochemistry of botulinum toxin type B. *Neurology.* 2000;55(Suppl 5):S22-S28.
7. Popoff MR, Marvaud JC, Raffestin S. [Mechanism of action and therapeutic uses of botulinum and tetanus neurotoxins]. *Ann Pharm Fr.* 2001;59(3):176-190.
8. Keller JE, Neale EA, Oyler G, et al. Persistence of botulinum neurotoxin action in cultured spinal cord cells. *FEBS Lett.* 1999;456(1):137-142.
9. Angaut-Petit D, Molgo J, Comello JX, et al. Terminal sprouting in mouse neuromuscular junctions poisoned with botulinum type-A toxin: morphological and electrophysiological features. *Neuroscience.* 1990;37(3):799-808.
10. Boni R, Kreyden OP, Burg G. Revival of the use of botulinum toxin: application in dermatology. *Dermatology.* 2000;200(4):287-291.
11. Edelstein C, Shorr N, Jacobs J, Balch K, Goldberg R. Oculoplastic experience with the cosmetic use of botulinum A exotoxin. *Dermatol Surg.* 1998;24(11):1208-1212.
12. Matarasso SL. Complications of botulinum A exotoxin for hyperfunctional lines. *Dermatol Surg.* 1998;24(11):1249-1254.
13. Carruthers JA, Lowe NJ, Menter MA, et al. A multicenter, double-blind, randomized, placebo-controlled study of the efficacy and safety of botulinum toxin type-A in the treatment of glabellar lines. *J Am Acad Dermatol.* 2002;46(6):840-849.

.

CHAPTER 3

Pertinent Facial Muscle Anatomy

William J. Lipham, MD, FACS

Since botulinum toxin exerts its effects by inactivating muscle contraction, it is essential for clinicians to be familiar with underlying facial muscle anatomy in order to obtain optimal results and avoid unnecessary complications. Facial muscle anatomy is complex and requires a thorough understanding of both agonist and antagonist muscles, whose relationship to one another must be appreciated prior to administering botulinum toxin. The purpose of this chapter is to review the relevant anatomy of the forehead, brow, and periocular region as well as the other muscles of the face and neck that are commonly treated with botulinum toxin. The muscles of the upper face that are commonly treated with botulinum toxin include the frontalis, procerus, corrugator/depressor supercilii complex, orbicularis oculi, and nasalis muscles. Patients with hemifacial spasm or Meige syndrome may also have spasm of the zygomaticus major and minor muscles of the mid face that require treatment. In the lower face, the perioral region may be treated by injecting small doses of botulinum toxin into the orbicularis oris at multiple sites and the depressor anguli oris while the neck may be treated by injecting the platysma muscle (Figure 3-1).

The Frontalis Muscle

The frontalis muscles are vertically oriented and form the anterior belly of the occipitofrontalis musculofacial complex (the occipitalis projects posteriorly). The frontalis arises from the galea aponeurotica near the coronal suture at the top of the skull and interdigitates with fibers of the procerus, corrugator, and orbicularis oculi muscles (Figure 3-2). The frontalis has no bony attachments, is closely attached to the underlying skin, and is separated by only a thin layer of superficial fascia. Contraction of this muscle group is responsible for elevation of the brow, which may induce horizontal or transverse wrinkles across the forehead (Figure 3-3).[1] Centrally, the frontalis muscle contains more fibrous connective tissue than the lateral regions and, therefore, typically requires less botulinum toxin.

The antagonists of the frontalis muscle are the central brow depressors, consisting of the procerus, corrugator, and depressor supercilii muscles, and the lateral depressor

Figure 3-1. The primary muscles of facial expression treated with botulinum toxin administration include the following: (A) frontalis; (B) corrugator and depressor supercilii complex; (C) orbicularis oculi; (D) procerus; (E) platysma; (F) nasalis; (G) orbicularis oris; (H) depressor anguli oris; (I) zygomaticus major; (J) zygomaticus minor. (Courtesy of Emerging Pharma, Inc.)

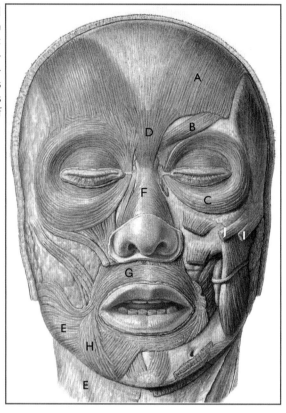

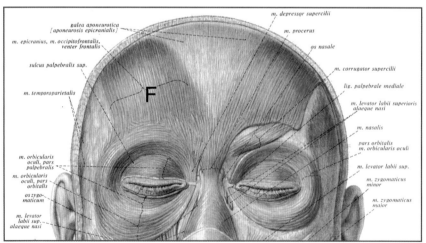

Figure 3-2. The frontalis muscle (F) arises from the galea aponeurotica near the coronal suture, inserts onto the superciliary ridge of the frontal bone, and interdigitates with fibers of the procerus, corrugator, depressor supercilii, and orbicularis oculi muscles. (Courtesy of Emerging Pharma, Inc.)

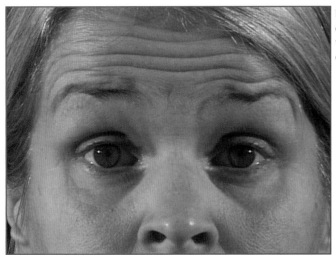

Figure 3-3. The frontalis muscle elevates the brows and creates transverse forehead lines when contracted.

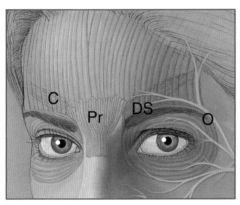

Figure 3-4. The brow depressors are the antagonist muscles of the frontalis muscle and include the following: (Pr) procerus muscle; (C) corrugator muscle; (DS) depressor supercilii; (O) superolateral portion of the preorbital orbicularis muscle, which is responsible for lateral brow depression. (Illustration by Lauren Shavell of Medical Imagery.)

of the brow, the superolateral portion of the preorbital orbicularis oculi (Figure 3-4).[2] Inactivation of the entire frontalis muscle will result in significant brow ptosis due to the unopposed action of these brow depressors. For this reason, it is important to discuss this agonist/antagonist relationship between the 2 muscle groups with patients who are interested in having their transverse brow lines treated but who do not desire treatment of their brow depressors. Optimal results with respect to brow height and contour are usually obtained with either low-dose treatment of the frontalis muscle or coadministration of botulinum toxin to both the frontalis muscle and brow depressors in order to equally weaken both muscle groups.

The Brow Depressors

As mentioned previously, the central brow depressors are composed of the procerus, corrugator, and depressor supercilii muscles.[3] In addition, the superolateral orbital portion of the orbicularis muscle is responsible for depressing the lateral aspect of the brow (see Figure 3-4). The procerus muscle originates from the lower portion of the nasal bone and inserts into the skin overlying the nasal root. It interdigitates with fibers of the orbicularis, frontalis, and corrugator muscles. Contraction of the procerus muscle induces

Figure 3-5. Contraction of the corrugator/depressor supercilii complex produces vertical glabellar furrows or "frown" lines.

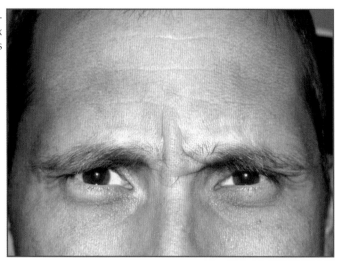

a transverse line at the nasal bridge as the muscle contracts vertically and centrally depresses the brow over the nasal bridge.[4] In contrast, the corrugator muscle, along with the depressor supercilii muscle, is responsible for the vertical glabellar furrows or frown lines that may develop medial to the brow cilia (Figure 3-5). The corrugator muscle lies deep to the procerus as well as the frontalis muscles. It originates from the superomedial aspect of the orbital rim just medial to the brow cilia. It then passes laterally through the galeal fat pad above the brow to insert into the superficial dermis within the central aspect of the eyebrow. The depressor supercilii muscle is located just below the corrugator muscle and similarly contributes to the creation of glabellar furrows or "frown" lines.[3] When botulinum toxin is administered into the region of the corrugator muscle, it also weakens the depressor supercilii as these muscles lie in close juxtaposition and can be conceptualized as a single functional entity.

It should be noted that the supratrochlear as well as the supraorbital neurovascular bundles emanate from the superomedial aspect of the orbit to provide sensation as well as a blood supply to the forehead and brow region. For this reason, it is important to palpate the supraorbital rim to appreciate the location of the supraorbital notch and thereby avoid injecting directly into the supraorbital bundle, which may injure the associated artery and nerves, resulting in pain and bruising.[5]

The lateral brow depressors consist of the superolateral aspect of the preorbital portion of the orbicularis oculi muscle. These fibers are typically located just below the lateral aspect of the brow cilia. Inactivation of this portion of the orbicularis muscle in association with inactivation of the central brow depressors can provide approximately 2 mm to 3 mm of brow elevation, which has been described as a "chemical browlift."[6] It is important to avoid injecting too deep in this area because the orbicularis muscle is relatively thin and inadvertent administration of botulinum toxin behind the orbital septum may induce a transient ptosis. Typically, a superficial injection technique in this area is the best approach.

The Orbicularis Oculi

The orbicularis muscle is a ring-like striated muscle sheet that lies just below the skin. It is separated from the overlying dermis by a fibroadipose layer that may be 4 mm to

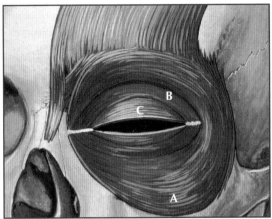

Figure 3-6. The orbicularis muscle is divided into the (A) preorbital, (B) preseptal, and (C) pretarsal portions based on both function and anatomy. (Reprinted from *Atlas of Clinical and Surgical Orbital Anatomy*, JJ Dutton, © 1994, with permission from Elsevier.)

6 mm thick underneath the brow region but that is less than 0.1 mm in thickness in the pretarsal portion of the eyelid where it terminates at the eyelid margin.[7] The orbicularis muscle is divided anatomically into 3 regions: the preorbital, preseptal, and pretarsal (Figure 3-6).

The preorbital portion of the orbicularis muscle arises from insertions on the frontal process of the maxillary bone in front of the anterior lacrimal crest and from the common medial canthal tendon. Its fibers pass around the orbital rim to form an elliptical shape that is continuous without interruption at the lateral commissure that inserts just below their original points of origin.

In contrast, the palpebral portion of the orbicularis muscle consists of 2 hemi-ellipses of muscle that are fixed medially and laterally at the medial and lateral canthal tendon complexes. While this portion forms a single anatomical unit, it is traditionally divided topographically into the preseptal and pretarsal orbicularis. The preseptal portion is positioned over the orbital septum in both the upper and lower eyelids. The preseptal orbicularis muscle appears to function largely by counteracting the opposing tone of the eyelid retractors. It also contributes to the lacrimal pump mechanism since it is associated medially with Horner's muscle of the lacrimal sac. The pretarsal orbicularis muscle originates from the superficial and deep portion of the medial canthal tendon complex. The superficial heads of the pretarsal orbicularis muscle insert into the anterior arm of the medial canthal tendon and run nearly parallel to the horizontal plane of the eyelid margin. The deep heads invest the canaliculi and are involved with the lacrimal pump mechanism.

Contraction of the lateral portion of the preseptal and preorbital portion of the orbicularis muscle causes the formation of "crow's feet" or "smile" lines (Figure 3-7).[8] These lines can be inactivated by injecting botulinum toxin into the preseptal and preorbital orbicularis muscle in the area just lateral to the orbital rim. Typically 2 to 3 injections are used to distribute botulinum toxin to this area. It is important to palpate the region of muscle contraction in order to inactivate the lateral orbicularis muscle. Care should be taken to avoid injecting within the orbital rim because this increases the likelihood of diffusion of the botulinum toxin behind the septum, which may induce ectropion or ptosis.

Patients with primary essential blepharospasm or hemifacial spasm may exhibit uncontrolled spasmodic contraction of the entire orbicularis muscle complex.[9] Essential blepharospasm is felt to arise from a central nervous system defect in the basal ganglion of the mid brain.[10] In contrast, hemifacial spasm is a disorder of the peripheral nervous system most commonly associated with irritation of the seventh cranial nerve after it exits

Figure 3-7. Contraction of the lateral portion of the preseptal and preorbital portion of the orbicularis oris muscle induces "crow's feet" or "smile" lines.

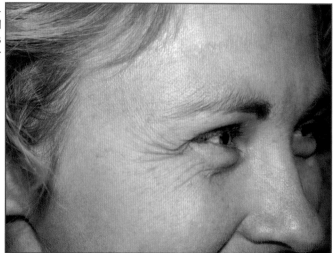

Figure 3-8. Contraction of the nasalis creates ridges on the nasal bridge that have been referred to as "bunny" lines.

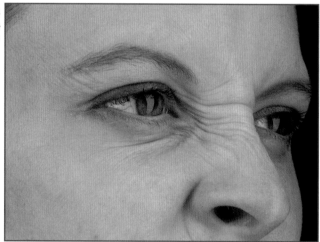

the brainstem. The spasm is felt to arise from irritation of the facial nerve by an adjacent artery that shares a common adventitial sheath.[11,12] As its name implies, this process is typically unilateral and may involve the orbicularis muscle as well as other muscles of facial expression, including the muscles of the mid face, lower face, and neck region.

The Nasalis

The nasalis or compressor naris muscle arises from the maxilla, and its fibers proceed upwards and medially, expanding into a thin aponeurosis that is continuous on the bridge of the nose with that of the muscle of the opposite side, and with the aponeurosis of the procerus muscle (see Figure 3-1). Contraction of the nasalis depresses the cartilaginous part of the nose and draws the ala toward the septum, creating ridges on the nasal bridge that have been referred to as "bunny" lines (Figure 3-8).

Zygomaticus Major and Minor

The zygomaticus major muscle originates along the inferolateral aspect of the orbital rim from the zygomatic bone, in front of the zygomaticotemporal suture, and descends obliquely and medially where it inserts into the angle of the mouth (see Figure 3-1). At its insertion near the mouth, it blends with the fibers of the orbicularis oris and depressor anguli oris, which act as its primary antagonists. Zygomaticus minor arises just medial and inferior to zygomaticus major and works in synergy with its larger lateral counterpart to form a functional complex. Contraction of the zygomaticus muscle complex draws the angle of the mouth backward and upward, as in laughing. This muscle is frequently involved in individuals with hemifacial spasm or Meige syndrome where its involuntary contraction can be disturbing to the patient as it elevates the lateral aspect of the upper lip and slightly opens the mouth.

The Orbicularis Oris

The orbicularis oris is not a simple sphincter muscle like the orbicularis oculi; it consists of numerous layers of muscle fibers surrounding the opening of the mouth that are oriented in many different directions. It is partially derived from the fibers of other facial muscles that are inserted into the lips and partly from fibers proper to the lips. Of the former, a considerable number are derived from the buccinator and form the deeper layers of the orbicularis. Some of the buccinator fibers—namely, those near the middle of the muscle, those arising from the maxilla passing to the lower lip, and those from the mandible to the upper lip—decussate at the angle of the mouth (Figure 3-9). The uppermost and lowermost fibers of the buccinator pass across the lips from side to side without decussation.

The proper fibers of the lips are oblique and pass from the under surface of the skin to the mucous membrane through the thickness of the lip. Finally, there are central fibers that connect the muscle with the maxilla and the septum of the nose superiorly and with the mandible inferiorly. In the upper lip these consist of the incisivus labii superioris (which arises from the alveolar border of the maxilla, opposite the lateral incisor tooth, and is continuous with the other muscles at the angle of the mouth) and the nasolabialis (which connects the upper lip to the back of the septum of the nose). The interval between the nasolabialis corresponds with the philtrum, which is the central depression seen on the lip beneath the nasal septum. The incisivus labii inferioris, a less complex structure, is present in the lower lip and arises from the mandible to intermingle with other muscles at the angle of the mouth.

The orbicularis oris in its ordinary action affects the direct closure of the lips; by its deep fibers, assisted by the oblique ones, it closely applies the lips to the alveolar arch. This is very important in keeping the lips in their proper position during mastication and pronunciation of words. The superficial portion, consisting principally of the decussating fibers, brings the lips together and also protrudes them forward in a "kissing" action. This pursing action of the superficial muscle fibers is what contributes to the formation of perioral rhytides or "smoker's" lines (Figure 3-10). It is important that small doses of botulinum toxin are administered to these superficial fibers only in order to avoid problems with mastication and pronunciation, which may occur if the deeper buccinator fibers are inactivated.

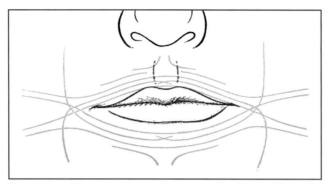

Figure 3-9. The orbicularis oris is partially derived from the buccinator, which forms the deeper layers of the orbicularis. The uppermost and lowermost fibers of the buccinator pass across the lips from side to side without decussation. The proper fibers of the lips are oblique and pass from the under surface of the skin to the mucous membrane, through the thickness of the lip. In the upper lip these consist of the incisivus labii superioris, which arises from the alveolar border of the maxilla and is continuous with the other muscles at the angle of the mouth, as well as the nasolabialis, which connects the upper lip to the back of the septum of the nose. The incisivus labii inferioris, a less complex structure, is present in the lower lip and arises from the mandible to intermingle with other muscles at the angle of the mouth.

Figure 3-10. Contraction of the superficial muscle fibers of the orbicularis oris contributes to the formation of perioral rhytides or "smoker's" lines.

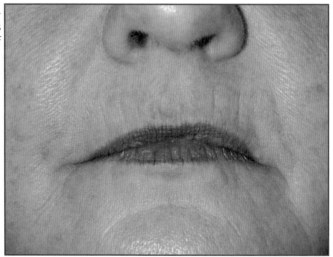

The Depressor Anguli

The triangularis or depressor anguli oris arises from the oblique line of the mandible and inserts, by a narrow fasciculus, into the angle of the mouth (Figure 3-11). It is continuous with the platysma at its origin and with the orbicularis oris at its insertion. Contraction of this muscle over time results in melomental folds or "marionette" lines, which may be treated with dermal filler agents or softened by injecting botulinum toxin directly into the depressor anguli oris muscle.

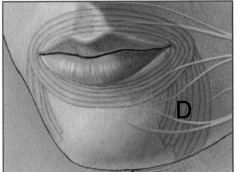

Figure 3-11. The triangularis or depressor anguli oris (D) arises from the oblique line of the mandible and inserts, by a narrow fasciculus, into the angle of the mouth. (Illustration by Lauren Shavell of Medical Imagery.)

The Platysma

The platysma is a broad sheet of muscle arising from the fascia of the pectoralis and the deltoid muscles. Its fibers cross the clavicle and extend obliquely and upward along the side of the neck (see Figure 3-1). The fibers then extend across the angle of the jaw and insert into the skin and subcutaneous tissue of the lower face as well as the muscles surrounding the angle and the lower part of the mouth, including the depressor anguli oris. With aging, the cervical neck skin loses its elasticity and the anterior portion of the platysmal muscle separates to form 2 diverging vertical bands. These bands contract and become more visible when the neck is animated (Figure 3-12). Botulinum toxin may be directly injected into these bands to reduce their appearance by weakening the force of contraction.

Summary

It is important that physicians have a sound fund of knowledge with respect to facial muscle anatomy before they implement botulinum toxin treatments into their clinical armamentarium. While this chapter provides a foundation in this regard, it is important to learn how these various muscle groups function in real life. This type of experience is best obtained by taking hands-on skills transfer courses or spending time with a practitioner who regularly performs botulinum toxin injections for a variety of indications.

References

1. Wieder JM, Moy RL. Understanding botulinum toxin: surgical anatomy of the frown, forehead, and periocular region. *Dermatol Surg.* 1998;24(11):1172-1174.
2. Dutton JJ. *Atlas of Clinical and Surgical Orbital Anatomy.* Philadelphia: WB Saunders; 1994.
3. Cook BE, Jr, Lucarelli MJ, Lemke BN. Depressor supercilii muscle: anatomy, histology, and cosmetic implications. *Ophthal Plast Reconstr Surg.* 2001;17(6):404-411.
4. Pribitkin EA, Greco TM, Goode RL, Keane WM. Patient selection in the treatment of glabellar wrinkles with botulinum toxin type A injection. *Arch Otolaryngol Head Neck Surg.* 1997;123(3):321-326.
5. Koch RJ, Troell RJ, Goode RL. Contemporary management of the aging brow and forehead. *Laryngoscope.* 1997;107(6):710-715.

Figure 3-12. Contraction of the platysma induces formation of platysmal bands that may be cosmetically undesirable. Botulinum toxin may be directly injected into these bands to reduce their appearance.

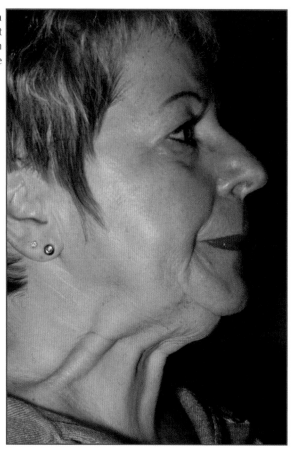

6. Frankel AS, Kamer FM. Chemical browlift. *Arch Otolaryngol Head Neck Surg.* 1998;124(3):321-323.
7. Harris CP, Alderson K, Nebeker J, Holds JB, Anderson RL. Histologic features of human orbicularis oculi treated with botulinum A toxin. *Arch Ophthalmol.* 1991;109(3):393-395.
8. Guerrissi J, Sarkissian P. Local injection into mimetic muscles of botulinum toxin A for the treatment of facial lines. *Ann Plast Surg.* 1997;39(5):447-453.
9. Borodic GE, Cozzolino D. Blepharospasm and its treatment, with emphasis on the use of botulinum toxin. *Plast Reconstr Surg.* 1989;83(3):546-554.
10. Dutton JJ, Buckley EG. Botulinum toxin in the management of blepharospasm. *Arch Neurol.* 1986;43(4):380-382.
11. Chen RS, Lu CS, Tsai CH. Botulinum toxin A injection in the treatment of hemifacial spasm. *Acta Neurol Scand.* 1996;94(3):207-211.
12. Cuevas C, Madrazo I, Magallon E, Zamorano C, Neri G, Reyes E. Botulinum toxin-A for the treatment of hemifacial spasm. *Arch Med Res.* 1995;26(4):405-408.

CHAPTER 4

Getting Started: Commercially Available Products, Basic Equipment and Supplies, Reconstitution and Dilution Recommendations, and Clinical Implementation

William J. Lipham, MD, FACS

Commercially Available Botulinum Toxin Agents

There are presently 3 commercially available products containing botulinum toxin for medical use in various parts of the world. Botulinum toxin type-A is commercially available as 2 preparations: BOTOX and Dysport (Figure 4-1). While BOTOX is available worldwide, Dysport is currently available in the European Union and Asia but is not approved for clinical use in the United States or Canada. In the United States, marketing and distribution of Dysport was initially sold to Inamed Aesthetics who changed the name of the compound to Reloxin. In 2006, Inamed was purchased by Allergan, the manufacturer of BOTOX and BOTOX Cosmetic. To avoid antitrust issues, Allergan is selling the marketing and distribution rights for Reloxin to an as-yet undisclosed competitor. Botulinum toxin type-B is currently approved for use in the United States and is commercially available as MYOBLOC (Figure 4-2). MYOBLOC is currently only available in the United States but will soon become available in Canada and Europe. It should be noted, however, that only BOTOX has received approval from the FDA for the reduction of glabellar furrows or "frown" lines. This approval for BOTOX does not extend to other cosmetic indications or applications, and when any of these preparations are used for cosmetic purposes in any other location, they are done so in an "off-label" fashion.

While both BOTOX and Dysport are sold as lyophilized powder that requires subsequent reconstitution with sterile saline, MYOBLOC is sold as an aqueous solution in a

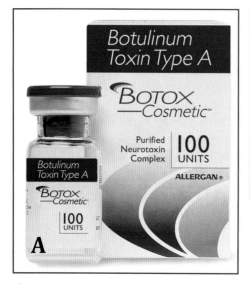
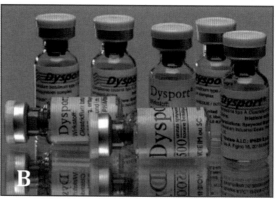

Figure 4-1. Botulinum toxin type-A preparations that are commercially available include (A) BOTOX and (B) Dysport. While BOTOX is available worldwide, Dysport is currently available in the European Union and Asia but is not approved for clinical use in the United States or Canada.

Figure 4-2. MYOBLOC, a purified form of botulinum toxin type-B, is currently only available in the United States but will soon become available in Canada and Europe. (Courtesy of Élan Pharmaceuticals.)

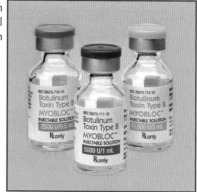

3.5-mL vial at a pH of 5.6. It is felt that this relatively acidic pH can be attributed to the increased discomfort that patients subjectively experience with MYOBLOC injections.[1] Each vial contains 5000 units of botulinum toxin type-B per mL in 0.05% human serum albumin, 0.01 mg sodium succinate, and 0.1 mg sodium chloride. Because it comes in a solution, reconstitution is not required and it should be refrigerated (2°C to 8°C) but never frozen. MYOBLOC can also be diluted with nonpreserved saline. However, any diluted portion should be used within 4 hours of dilution since the saline contains no preservatives. MYOBLOC is reported to have a shelf life of 36 months if refrigerated and 9 months at room temperature.

In a study comparing MYOBLOC and BOTOX for the treatment of lateral canthal rhytides, MYOBLOC was shown to cause slightly more discomfort upon injection, specifically a sensation of "tightness" of the treated area. A quicker onset of action and a briefer duration of muscle paralysis were also associated with MYOBLOC, which has an onset of 48 hours and usually lasts 6 to 8 weeks.[2] An advantage of MYOBLOC appears to be its shelf life, which allows the practitioner more flexibility in scheduling patients for treatment because patients do not have to be grouped together.

Dosing of botulinum toxin agents is described in units of biological activity (units). For all of these compounds, 1 units is defined as the amount of neurotoxin complex that is lethal in 50% of female, Swiss-Webster mice after a single intraperitoneal injection (mouse LD50). While the definition of a unit of toxin is similar to all 3 compounds, the formulation as well as the methods in which the lethality tests are performed by the different manufacturers vary significantly, resulting in discrepancies with respect to the potency of a single unit of botulinum toxin between the 3 manufacturers. Unfortunately, this results in a lack of uniformity between the 3 products with respect to dosing. A review of the literature reveals that unit doses of Dysport range from 3 to 4 times higher than equivalent doses of BOTOX when used to treat similar conditions.[3,4] In contrast, the unit doses of MYOBLOC are 50 to 100 times higher than those typically seen with BOTOX.[5] To compensate for this difference, each manufacturer produces vials that contain different unit quantities between manufacturers. For example, each vial of BOTOX contains 100 BOTOX units while Dysport is supplied with 500 Dysport units per vial. MYOBLOC is supplied as an aqueous solution at a concentration of 5000 MYOBLOC units per milliliter with 2500-unit, 5000-unit, and 10,000-unit vials available.

In light of these differences, it is absolutely crucial that the commercial product be identified when discussing the dose of botulinum toxin. Utilizing Dysport or MYOBLOC at BOTOX doses will result in little or no clinical effect while treatment with BOTOX utilizing Dysport or MYOBLOC dosing regimens could result in profound weakness and even potentially serious systemic side effects. Therefore, it is imperative that the agent utilized be clearly described whenever dosing and administration are discussed.[6,7]

It has been the author's experience that botulinum toxin type-A compounds are easier to incorporate into clinical practice since they have good dose correlations and are less painful when injected. At present, I only use botulinum toxin type-B or MYOBLOC in selected patients with blepharospasm or hemifacial spasm who no longer respond well to botulinum toxin type-A therapy. Typically, these are individuals who have received BOTOX for more than 5 to 10 years and have subsequently developed neutralizing antibodies to botulinum toxin type-A that reduce its clinical effect.[7] I have found that these same patients, however, still respond to botulinum toxin type-B, and I limit my usage of this compound to this particular clinical indication. As such, I will limit discussions for the remainder of this text to Dysport and BOTOX, which are widely used botulinum toxin type-A preparations.

Essential Equipment and Supplies

It is essential for practitioners to obtain the basic supplies that are necessary for performing botulinum toxin treatments. The basic equipment includes the following (Figure 4-3):

* 3-cc syringe with 25-gauge needle for reconstitution of botulinum toxin
* Vial of sterile, nonpreserved normal saline for injection
* Alcohol wipes
* Gauze pads
* 30-gauge needles for injection
* 1-cc tuberculin syringes
* Ice pack or frozen gel packs for anesthesia

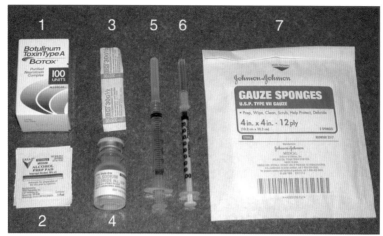

Figure 4-3. Basic supplies required for BOTOX injection treatments include the following: (1) vial of botulinum toxin; (2) alcohol wipes; (3) 30-gauge needles for injection; (4) vial of sterile, nonpreserved normal saline for injection; (5) 3-cc syringe with 25-gauge needle for reconstitution of botulinum toxin; (6) 1-cc tuberculin syringes; (7) gauze pads.

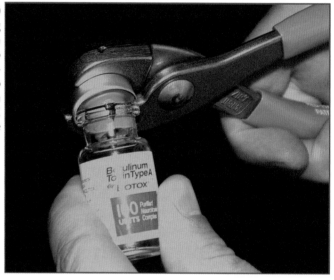

Figure 4-4. Twenty dollars to $40 is lost every time a vial containing 0.1 mL to 0.2 mL of botulinum toxin is discarded with the cap in place. To avoid this unnecessary waste, I recommend using a decapper device to safely and easily remove the cap from the vial. Decappers for both BOTOX and Dysport may be obtained online at www.kebbyindustries.com

❖ Some individuals also recommend lidocaine 4% topical anesthetic cream or Emla® cream (Abraxis Pharmaceuticals Products, Schaumburg, Ill) as a topical anesthetic, but I find these messy and prefer cold therapy for topical anesthesia

In addition, I have found with experience that it is very difficult to remove the final 0.1 mL of botulinum toxin solution from the vial unless the cap is removed. Unfortunately, the cap is held firmly in place and is very difficult to take off without inducing a potential injury. It should be noted that a practitioner loses $20 to $40 every time a vial containing 0.1 mL to 0.2 mL of botulinum toxin is discarded. To prevent this, I recommend using a Plier decapper device (Kebby Industries Inc, Rockfield, Ill) to safely and easily remove the vial cap (Figure 4-4). Decappers for both BOTOX and Dysport vials may be obtained online at www.kebbyindustries.com depending on the type of botulinum toxin used, as the size of the vials are different. This handy device rapidly pays for itself because it eliminates the problem of losing valuable botulinum toxin that cannot be removed from the vial if the cap is allowed to remain in place.

To streamline the treatment session, it is helpful to have a nurse or clinical assistant reconstitute the botulinum toxin while you evaluate the patient. Suggestions for reconstituting both BOTOX and Dysport are described in the next section.

Reconstitution, Dilution, and Storage Considerations

There are several underlying principles and guidelines that should be followed with respect to the reconstitution, dilution, and handling of these compounds. BOTOX and BOTOX Cosmetic are identical products that differ only by their product names and marketing strategies. For the remainder of this book, BOTOX will be used to describe both these compounds. The vials contain a freeze-dried material and should be stored in a freezer at or below −5°C. Each vial contains 100 units of botulinum toxin type-A, 0.5 mg of human albumin, and 0.9 mg of sodium chloride. According to the manufacturer, 0.9% sterile, nonpreserved saline solution should be added to the vial prior to use. Alternatively, a recent study demonstrated reduced pain in patients undergoing injections with botulinum toxin type-A prepared with a 0.9% preservative-containing bacteriostatic saline. Preservative-free and preservative-containing preparations appear to be equally efficacious. The bacteriostatic preservative benzyl alcohol has anesthetic properties, which likely account for the difference in discomfort levels.[8]

Dysport, like BOTOX, is supplied in a lyophilized form and, therefore, must be reconstituted with sterile saline prior to use. The manufacturers recommend that Dysport should be reconstituted with sterile, nonpreserved saline solution and stored at 2°C to 8°C (refrigerator temperature). In addition to the study by Alam et al,[8] Garcia and Fulton reported equivalent success with preserved saline and also note that patients describe reduced discomfort during the injections, which they attribute to the fact that preserved saline is pH buffered.[9] In my practice, I have switched from using sterile, nonpreserved saline to bacteriostatic saline to reconstitute botulinum toxin since it does appear to reduce the pain of injections.

Both BOTOX and Dysport are very potent, but fragile, and should not be agitated or shaken because the protein can become denatured and rendered completely ineffective. According to the manufacturers, BOTOX is stable for 4 hours before it should be discarded, while Dysport is reported to be stable for 8 hours after reconstitution. During the reconstitution period, the solution should be stored in a refrigerator (2°C to 8°C). One study showed no degradation in the potency of BOTOX when refrigerated and used within 30 days,[9] while another showed a reduction to 50% efficacy after 7 days and minimal efficacy after 14 days.[3] In general, most practitioners use the reconstituted BOTOX within 1 to 7 days before discarding; however, neither manufacturer recommends this practice. It is the author's own personal experience as well as that of other practitioners that a useful guideline is to utilize or discard either compound within 24 hours after reconstitution.

RECONSTITUTING BOTOX

A review of the literature with regard to BOTOX reveals that dilutions ranging from 2.5 units/mL to 100 units/mL have been employed.[3,10,11] Most practitioners, however, use between 25 units/mL to 100 units/mL.[7] It has been the author's experience that using a

Table 4-1

BOTOX Reconstitution

Volume per Vial (mL)	Units per 0.1 cc	Units per 0.05 cc
1	10	5
2	5	2.5
4	2.5	1.25

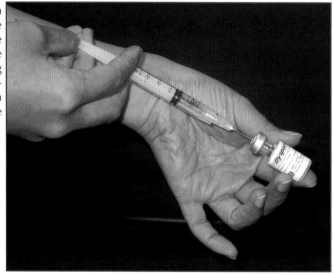

Figure 4-5. Care should be taken to hold onto the plunger of the 3-cc syringe when reconstituting the lyophilized botulinum toxin because excessive turbulence from injecting the solution rapidly into the container may dissociate the light chain from the heavy chain and render the molecule inactive.

concentration of 50 units/mL or 2 mL of sterile, nonpreserved normal saline per 100-units vial provides an excellent volume of distribution to obtain the desired clinical effect and provides a sufficient volume that makes injections easier to perform. While BOTOX may be reconstituted with 1 mL of sterile, nonpreserved saline to yield a concentration of 10 units/0.1 cc, it is more difficult to inject the proper volume with a 1-cc syringe because most sites will require 0.05 mL, which is somewhat difficult to accurately administer. Different individuals will find a particular concentration that works best in their hands, and a table is provided to produce a variety of dilutions for BOTOX (Table 4-1). I prefer to follow the manufacturer's recommendation and use a 3-cc syringe to reconstitute the lyophilized BOTOX with 2.5 mL of normal saline to provide a final concentration of approximately 4 units per 0.1 cc for cosmetic indications. For functional purposes, I typically use either 2.0 mL of saline for reconstitution, which yields an injection concentration of 5 units/0.1 mL. For the sake of this text, I will discuss BOTOX doses using the aforementioned dilution recommendations. If you treat both functional and cosmetic patients with the same vial of BOTOX, however, it may be easier in practice to use the same volume for both indications.

It should be noted that the sterile saline should be added slowly to the vial when reconstituting BOTOX. Care should be taken to hold onto the plunger of the syringe as it enters the vial since the lyophilized powder is maintained in a vacuum (Figure 4-5). A 25-gauge needle on a 3-cc syringe should be used for reconstituting the lyophilized powder with

Table 4-2

Dose-Volume Equivalency of BOTOX and Dysport

	BOTOX	*Dysport*
Vial contents	Type-A—100 units	Type-A—500 units
Reconstitution volume	2.5 mL	4.0 mL
Injection concentration	4 units/0.1 cc	12.5 units/0.1 cc

sterile, nonpreserved saline. If the normal saline is allowed to enter the vial rapidly, it will create significant turbulence, causing the light chains and heavy chains to disassociate and will render the botulinum toxin inactive. In addition, the contents of the vial should never be shaken, but instead be gently rotated or swirled to mix the solution.

RECONSTITUTING DYSPORT

Currently, the manufacturers of Dysport recommend diluting each vial with 2.5 cc of sterile, nonpreserved saline. This provides a solution with a concentration of 20 units/ 0.1 cc, which yields a 4:1 ratio when compared to an equivalent volume of BOTOX. At present, there are conflicting reports that describe the ratio of Dysport units to BOTOX units, ranging from 3:1 to 4:1.[3,4,12] While this dose regimen appears well founded for the treatment of functional disorders where larger doses of Dysport may be required, I have developed a slightly different dilution profile for cosmetic use.

For aesthetic purposes, I prefer to use Dysport at a concentration of 12.5 units/0.1 cc, as this provides a closer dose equivalent to BOTOX for a similar injection volume.[4] It has been the author's experience while working with Dysport in Asia that approximately 3 Dysport units are clinically equivalent to 1 BOTOX unit for cosmetic purposes. These observations are consistent with a randomized, double-blinded study that was performed to determine the dose equivalency of Dysport and BOTOX for the treatment of cervical dystonia.[4]

Since there are 500 units in each vial of Dysport, dose-volume equivalency with respect to BOTOX may be obtained by diluting each Dysport vial with 4.0 mL of sterile, nonpreserved saline (Table 4-2). I find this practice makes it easier to transfer between Dysport and BOTOX because the same treatment volumes will induce a similar clinical effect.

In summary, dilution of Dysport with 2.5 mL of saline will yield a stronger solution, which may be beneficial when treating larger muscle groups for spastic disorders, while dilution with 4.0 mL will yield a solution that more closely correlates to BOTOX that has been reconstituted with 2.5 mL of saline.

STORAGE

Both BOTOX and Dysport are provided as lyophilized powders that must be stored at reduced temperatures. BOTOX is supplied in a 100-units vial and must be stored at a temperature below 5°C, which is equivalent to temperatures obtained in a conventional freezer. In contrast, Dysport may be stored as a lyophilized powder at 2°C to 8°C, which corresponds to refrigeration temperatures. Following reconstitution, both compounds should be stored at refrigerator temperatures and never should be put in the freezer or kept at room temperature.

Figure 4-6. Reclining examination chair for BOTOX injections. The patient is reclined about 25 to 30 degrees from the vertical upright position to facilitate proper injection technique.

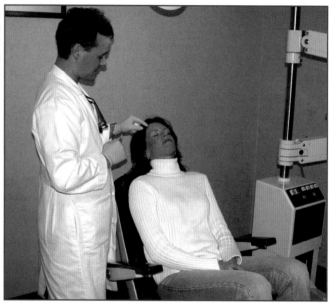

Clinical Implementation

I have found that it is easiest to treat patients in a reclining examination chair as compared to a conventional chair or bed since this allows the physician to adjust the height and angle of the patient. Injections are usually administered with the patient reclining at an approximately 25-degree to 30-degree angle from a vertically upright position (Figure 4-6). If the patient has blepharospasm, hemifacial spasm, or Meige syndrome, the frequency and intensity of the spasm are graded on a 1- to 4-point scale and the treatment plan is mapped out on a clinical exam sheet (Figure 4-7). The treatment plan documents the dose and locations for each injection site. This can then be referred to on subsequent visits to adjust the location and dosage of the injections to obtain the desired result. A consent form that the patient must review and sign before each injection session is on the reverse side of the BOTOX injection form (Figure 4-8). To enhance patient flow in the clinic, I provide the patient with his or her consent/treatment form when he or she checks in at the front desk so he or she has time to review it in the waiting room. Once the patient has reviewed the consent form, he or she is then able to ask me any questions he or she may have prior to signing the form. I make sure that both my nurse and myself personally verify that the consent form is signed before I fill out the treatment plan.

Once the patient has signed the consent form and the total dose of botulinum toxin has been calculated, the individual who is going to administer the botulinum toxin draws the appropriate amount from the vial into a 1-cc syringe with a 25-gauge needle. It is important to note that an additional 0.05 mL is typically withdrawn to allow for the volume of solution that is typically lost in the hub of the syringe needle. While some authors advocate the use of hubless insulin syringes, I have found that the 30-gauge needle becomes rather dull after it has been inserted through the rubber stopper of the botulinum toxin vial. Unfortunately, a dull needle makes the injections more painful, which may negatively impact patient satisfaction and limit return visits. For this reason, I use a 1-cc syringe with a plunger that enters the hub to minimize the loss of botulinum toxin. The 25-gauge needle is removed from the 1-cc syringe and a separate 30-gauge needle is then used for the injections.

BOTOX® TREATMENT FORM

Patient Name:
Acct # :
Date of Service:

Pre Injection Spasm:

LIDS: OD ___   OS ___

BROWS: R ___   L ___

FACE: R ___   L ___

NECK: R ___   L ___

0 = None
1 = Increased Blink
2 = Tolerable Flutter
3 = Mildly Incapacitating Spasm
4 = Severely Incapacitating Spasm

Injection No.   _____
Lot No./ Vial No. _____

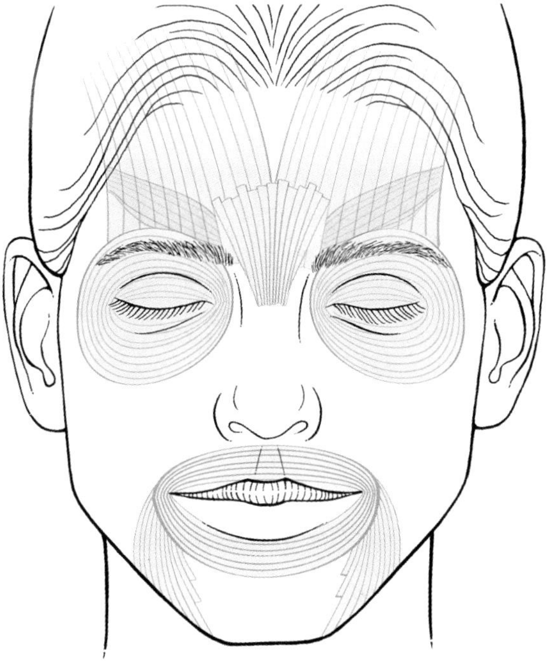

Dilution:

1.25 U/0.1ml   2.5 U/0.1ml   5.0 U/0.1ml   10U/0.1ml

Total Units – Lids/ Brow   R_____   L_____
Total Units – Crows feet   R_____   L_____
Total Units – Forehead   _____
Total Units – Other   _____   _____

        TOTAL UNITS   _____   TOTAL COST_____

Diagnosis: _____

Plan: _____

_____
Physician's Signature

Figure 4-7. Clinical exam sheet for BOTOX patients. The form provides a pictorial account of the injection pattern and dose received as well as the grade of spasm intensity and frequency. Informed consent is printed on the reverse side of this form. (Illustration by Lauren Shavell of Medical Imagery.)

Consent for Use of BOTOX®

BOTOX® is a brand name for botulinum toxin type A, a neurotoxin that blocks muscle contraction by temporarily inactivating the nerves that control them. The effects of BOTOX® become apparent 2-5 days after the injection and generally last 3-4 months. The FDA has approved the use of BOTOX® to treat facial dystonias (spasms), strabismus (crossed eyes) and to soften facial rhytids (wrinkles). There may be alternatives to BOTOX® including medicines or surgery.

Unwanted side effects of BOTOX® include but are not limited to;

- Local bleeding
- Bruising
- Undercorrection (not enough effect) or overcorrection (too much effect)
- Facial asymmetry (one side looks different than the other)
- Paralysis of a nearby muscle leading to: droopy eyelid, double vision, inability to close the eye, difficulty whistling or drinking from a straw
- Generalized weakness
- Permanent loss of muscle tone with repeated injection
- Flu-like syndrome
- Development of antibodies to BOTOX®
- Infection

BOTOX® contains Human-derived albumin and carries a theoretic risk of virus transmission. There have been no reports of disease transmission through BOTOX®. If you are pregnant, nursing or are allergic to albumin (eggs), you should not receive injections. Patients taking aminoglycoside antibiotics, or with Eaton-Lambert syndrome, Lou Gehrig's disease or myasthenia gravis should not have BOTOX®.

••

I understand the above and have had the risks, benefits and alternatives explained to me. I give my informed consent for BOTOX® injections today.

_____   _____
Patient Signature   Date

Figure 4-8. Informed consent form for BOTOX administration. The form should be signed by the patient and physician prior to planning the injection dose and pattern of distribution.

While the calculations and the amount of botulinum toxin are being determined by the physician and drawn up into the 1-cc syringes, the assistant provides the patient with a cold gel pack to provide topical anesthesia. The patient is asked to apply the gel pack to the area being treated for approximately 1 to 2 minutes to achieve adequate pain relief (Figure 4-9). The gel pack is then removed and the injection sites are cleansed with alcohol prep pads to prevent cutaneous infection (Figure 4-10). The injections are administered as described in detail in the following chapters, and light pressure is applied to each injection site with a gauze pad. The syringe is held in the injector's dominant hand while

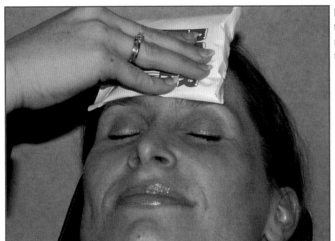

Figure 4-9. A cold pack is applied to the area to be treated for approximately 1 minute to provide adequate topical anesthesia prior to injection.

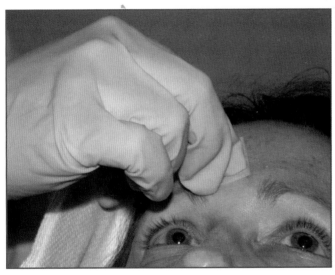

Figure 4-10. Alcohol wipes are used to remove any makeup, cleanse the skin, and reduce the risk of cutaneous infection prior to injection.

the gauze pad is held in the injector's nondominant hand at all times. If any pinpoint bleeding is noted following the initial injection, pressure is immediately applied to the area to reduce the risk of post-treatment bruising or ecchymosis (Figure 4-11). I typically give 2 to 3 injections in sequence to treat a local functional unit and then give the patient a moment to recover (approximately 15 to 30 seconds) before moving on and injecting the next region. Once the treatment is complete, an additional gauze pad is given to the patient so that he or she may dab any pinpoint bleeders that may develop after he or she leaves the office.

While some clinicians recommend that patients actively contract the muscle areas that have been treated, a thorough understanding of the mechanism of action of botulinum toxin would reveal that receptor-mediated binding is not dependent upon muscle contraction. In light of this, I do not feel that patients need to perform facial muscle exercises following injections. I do, however, recommend that patients refrain from vigorous aerobic activity for at least 24 hours following their initial botulinum toxin injection to prevent unwanted diffusion of botulinum toxin into adjacent muscle groups, which may be facilitated by increased blood flow.

Figure 4-11. After an injection has been performed, light pressure is applied with a gauze pad to reduce the risk of post-treatment bruising or ecchymosis.

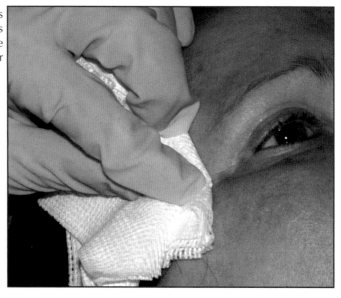

The patient is also instructed to observe his or her muscle activity over the next 3 to 4 days and is reminded that he or she will not see a treatment effect for at least a similar period of time. He or she is similarly instructed to follow up for retreatment in approximately 3 to 4 months or once it is felt that his or her muscle activity has returned to approximately 75% of its original strength. I also have my administrative assistant send out a reminder letter (in a sealed envelope to maintain confidentiality) to all of my botulinum toxin patients 3 months after their treatment to remind them that they may want to consider returning for an additional treatment.

References

1. Ramirez AL, Reeck J, Maas CS. Botulinum toxin type-B (MyoBloc) in the management of hyperkinetic facial lines. *Otolaryngol Head Neck Surg.* 2002;126(5):459-467.
2. Matarasso SL. Complications of botulinum A exotoxin for hyperfunctional lines. *Dermatol Surg.* 1998;24(11):1249-1254.
3. Lowe NJ. Botulinum toxin type-A for facial rejuvenation: United States and United Kingdom perspectives. *Dermatol Surg.* 1998;24(11):1216-1218.
4. Odergren T, Hjaltason S, Kaakkola S, et al. A double blind, randomized, parallel group study to investigate the dose equivalence of Dysport and BOTOX in the treatment of cervical dystonia. *J Neurol Neurosurg Psychiatry.* 1998;64(1):6-12.
5. Lew MF. Review of the FDA-approved uses of botulinum toxins, including data suggesting efficacy in pain reduction. *Clin J Pain.* 2002;18(6 Suppl):S142-S146.
6. Klein AW. Dilution and storage of botulinum toxin. *Dermatol Surg.* 1998;24(11):1179-1180.
7. Siatkowski RM, Tyutyunikov A, Biglan AW, et al. Serum antibody production to botulinum A toxin. *Ophthalmology.* 1993;100(12):1861-1866.
8. Alam M, Dover JS, Arndt KA. Pain associated with injection of botulinum A exotoxin reconstituted using isotonic sodium chloride with and without preservative: a double-blind, randomized controlled trial. *Arch Dermatol.* 2002;138:510-514.
9. Garcia A, Fulton JE, Jr. Cosmetic denervation of the muscles of facial expression with botulinum toxin: a dose-response study. *Dermatol Surg.* 1996;22(1):39-43.

10. Bulstrode NW, Grobbelaar AO. Long-term prospective follow-up of botulinum toxin treatment for facial rhytides. *Aesthetic Plast Surg.* 2002;26(5):356-359.
11. Carruthers A, Carruthers J. Clinical indications and injection technique for the cosmetic use of botulinum A exotoxin. *Dermatol Surg.* 1998;24(11):1189-1194.
12. Nussgens Z, Roggenkamper P. Comparison of two botulinum-toxin preparations in the treatment of essential blepharospasm. *Graefes Arch Clin Exp Ophthalmol.* 1997;235(4):197-199.

CHAPTER 5

Treatment of Blepharospasm, Meige Syndrome, and Hemifacial Spasm

William J. Lipham, MD, FACS

BOTOX was first approved by the US FDA in December 1989 for the treatment of strabismus and blepharospasm as well as other spastic disorders of the facial nerve, including hemifacial spasm and Meige syndrome in patients over the age of 12 years. In December 2000, BOTOX also received approval for the treatment of cervical dystonia, a neurological movement disorder causing severe neck and shoulder contractions. While all of these conditions are felt to be distinct entities with respect to their etiology, they are often grouped together as facial movement disorders. This chapter will review the pathophysiology and treatment of these facial movement disorders. The evaluation and treatment of strabismus, however, will be covered in a separate chapter. It should also be noted that while the author has considerable experience treating these movement disorders with BOTOX, he has significantly less experience with Dysport and will, therefore, make reference to BOTOX doses for the purposes of this chapter.

Pathophysiology

Blepharospasm or benign essential blepharospasm (BEB) is an idiopathic bilateral disorder characterized by episodic, involuntary contraction of the orbicularis oculi muscles, causing uncontrolled eyelid closure. Although the cause is unknown, the development of essential blepharospasm has been associated with radiologically demonstrated unilateral and bilateral thalamic lesions, bilateral basal ganglia lesions, and unilateral cerebellar and mesencephalic lesions. It usually begins as a mild and infrequent process but may progress to cause functional blindness (Figure 5-1).[1-8]

In contrast, hemifacial spasm and Meige syndrome are felt to arise from irritation of the seventh nerve or facial nerve after it exits the brainstem.[9-14] Since this process is typically unilateral, the spasm usually involves only one side of the facial musculature (Figure 5-2).[15] This is classically described as being caused by irritation of the peripheral facial nerve by an adjacent artery that shares a common adventitial sheath.[16-19] Microvascular decompression via a Jannetta procedure remains the only surgical solution for hemifacial

Figure 5-1. Blepharospasm is characterized by bilateral symmetric involuntary spasm of the eyelids that is felt to be due to a defect in the basal ganglion of the midbrain.

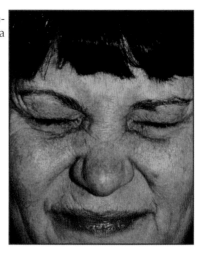

Figure 5-2. Hemifacial spasm is felt to be caused by irritation of the facial or seventh cranial nerve, resulting in unilateral contraction of the facial musculature.

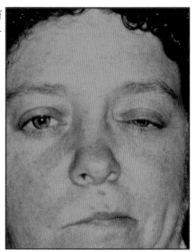

spasm or Meige syndrome.[20] This is a neurosurgical intervention in which the common adventitial sheath surrounding the artery and nerve is surgically released. A neurosurgical sponge is then placed between the offending artery and nerve to prevent nerve irritation, which induces spastic contraction of the facial musculature. While this treatment has an excellent success profile, it does expose the patient to a neurosurgical procedure with the associated risk of permanent facial paresis.

Aside from botulinum toxin injections, the only nonsurgical treatment for either of these conditions has consisted of central nervous system depressants, such as Valium® (Roche, Nutley, NJ) and Klonopin® (Roche). These drugs exert their effect by depressing the central nervous system thereby decreasing the spontaneous firing rate of the facial nerve, which in turn reduces involuntary orbicularis muscle contraction. Unfortunately, both of these medications are considerably sedating and are not viable long-term treatment options since they limit most individuals' activities of daily living.

Blepharospasm

Botulinum toxin is probably the single most effective treatment for patients with primary essential blepharospasm or BEB. When evaluating a patient with blepharospasm, it is important to obtain a complete medical history and determine the duration that he or she has had the condition. A recent diagnosis may indicate some variability with regard to the frequency and intensity of the condition, while chronicity may suggest a more stable course. In order to distinguish primary essential blepharospasm or BEB from a secondary form of blepharospasm (such as an aqueous tear deficiency), it is important to perform a complete eye examination to rule out keratitis sicca or any other ocular surface disorder (such as an allergy) that may incite blinking in an effort to alleviate ocular discomfort.

It is also important to discuss with patients how their spasm affects their normal activities of daily living. While some individuals may have very mild blepharospasm that does not induce significant functional difficulty, others may have such severe blepharospasm that they are unable to keep their eyes open for greater than 50% of the time, making driving and other visually demanding tasks difficult, if not impossible, to perform. It is also useful to ask if there are any factors that aggravate their symptoms or make their spasm increase in frequency or severity. These precipitating events typically include exposure to bright light or other less well-defined factors such as stress, which appears to play a significant role in patients with primary essential blepharospasm or BEB.

Once secondary causes such as an aqueous tear deficiency or ocular surface disease have been ruled out with a complete eye examination, a diagnosis of primary essential blepharospasm or BEB is further established by asking the patient if he or she is capable of reducing the spasm with any form of behavior modification. Many patients with primary essential blepharospasm or BEB will describe that they are able to decrease both the frequency and intensity of their spasms by singing, whistling, or forcefully elevating their eyebrows while those with underlying secondary causes of blepharospasm will not.

While the examining physician discusses these various historical points, it is important to simultaneously observe and evaluate the patient in order to grade the overall frequency and intensity of the spasm. The frequency and intensity of the spasm are individually graded on a 1-to-4 point scale with 1 representing mild frequency or intensity and 4 representing severe or incapacitating frequency or intensity. While this grading scheme is highly subjective and variable, it should be relatively consistent for each physician observer and should be used as the primary factor in determining which muscles are involved as well as establish the proper dosage for treatment and sites of injection.

TREATMENT OF MILD BLEPHAROSPASM

For individuals with a mild to moderate amount of blepharospasm, periocular injections are typically all that is required to control the spasm. As noted previously, the patient's spasm is evaluated and the involved muscle groups are identified. Typical initial doses consist of 2.5 units of BOTOX injected into the medial and lateral aspect of the upper eyelid at the level of the upper eyelid crease (Figure 5-3). These injections are performed to inactivate the pretarsal and preseptal orbicularis muscle of the upper eyelid. Since the skin in this location is only 60 µm in depth, it is important to insert the needle just below the skin surface and administer this injection subcutaneously in order to avoid inactivating the levator muscle, which lies immediately beneath the orbicularis muscle and septum.

The lateral aspect of the orbicularis oculi muscle is typically treated with 3 injections. The first injection is positioned at the lateral canthus, and the second and third injections

Figure 5-3. Treatment of mild to moderate blepharospasm: Injection of the pretarsal and preseptal portions of the orbicularis muscle. Typical initial doses consist of 2.5 units of BOTOX to the medial and lateral aspect of the upper eyelid along the eyelid crease. Since the skin is only 60 μm thick in this region, the injection is given subcutaneously to avoid penetrating the underlying septum and inducing ptosis of the upper eyelid.

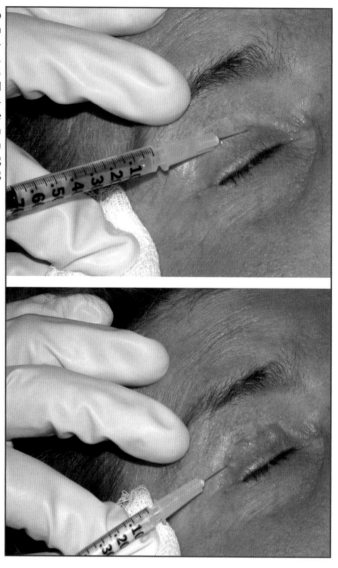

are positioned approximately 5 mm to 7 mm superior and inferior to the lateral canthal injection site (Figure 5-4). The superior and inferior injections typically consist of 5 units of BOTOX while 2.5 units to 5 units of BOTOX may be administered to the lateral canthal injection site (Figure 5-5).

If the lower lid is also involved in the spastic process, an additional lower lid injection may be performed approximately 1 cm inferior and lateral to the inferior punctum to inactivate the orbicularis muscle of the lower eyelid. Care must be taken here to avoid injecting too deep into the subcutaneous tissue because this may inactivate the inferior oblique muscle and induce diplopia. Care should also be taken to avoid injecting botulinum toxin close to the lower eyelid margin, which may inadvertently induce medial ectropion and epiphora. To avoid these complications, it is safest to start with an initial dose of 2.5 units of BOTOX to this area, realizing that the dose may be titrated upwards in subsequent injection sessions as indicated by the frequency and intensity of spasm.

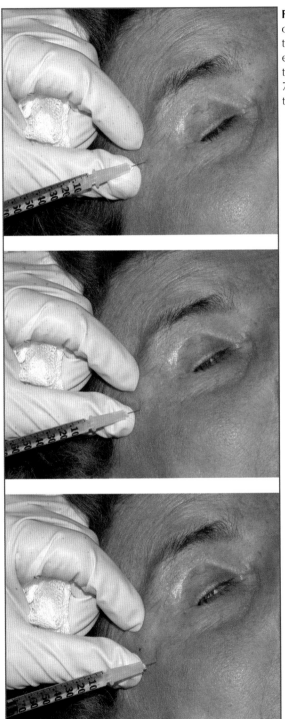

Figure 5-4. The lateral aspect of the orbicularis oculi muscle is typically treated with 3 injections. The first injection is positioned at the lateral canthus, and the second and third injections are positioned approximately 5 mm to 7 mm superior and inferior to the lateral canthal injection site.

Figure 5-5. Treatment of mild to moderate blepharospasm: Injection sites marked with a black "X" indicate regions that would typically receive 5 units of BOTOX while those marked with a gray "O" are regions that may be treated with either 2.5 or 5 units of BOTOX depending on the frequency and intensity of spasm. (Illustration by Lauren Shavell of Medical Imagery.)

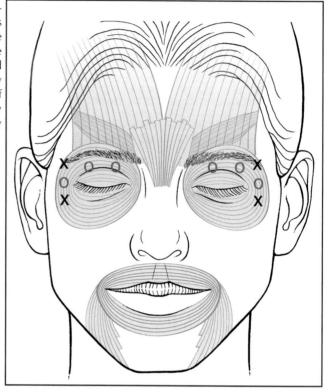

TREATMENT OF MODERATE TO SEVERE BLEPHAROSPASM

For patients with moderate to severe blepharospasm, additional areas outside of the orbicularis oculi muscle may need to be treated to completely inactivate the spasm. In a large number of patients with BEB, the central brow depressor muscles are frequently involved and may be more apparent in those with moderate to severe blepharospasm. These individuals are treated in a fashion similar to patients with mild to moderate blepharospasm, but they may also require an additional 2.5 units of BOTOX in the central aspect of the upper eyelid crease for a total of 7.5 units of BOTOX per eyelid (Figure 5-6). In addition, they usually require variable inactivation of the glabellar region that typically involves a dosing profile similar to that used for cosmetic purposes but is titrated according to the amount of muscle activity that is observed. Usually 20 to 25 units of BOTOX are required to limit the activity of the central brow depressors with 5 units administered to the procerus muscle and 7.5 to 10 units to each corrugator/depressor supercilii muscle complex (Figure 5-7). Since the superolateral aspect of the preorbital orbicularis oculi muscle may also be involved in brow depression and contribute to blepharospasm, an additional injection of 2.5 to 5 units of BOTOX placed below the lateral brow hairs may also improve their clinical response.

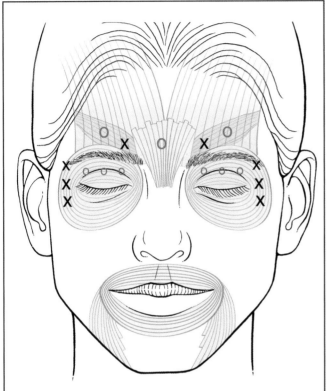

Figure 5-6. Treatment of moderate to severe blepharospasm: Injection sites marked with a black "X" indicate regions that would typically receive 5 units of BOTOX while those marked with a gray "O" are regions that may be treated with either 2.5 or 5 units of BOTOX depending on the frequency and intensity of spasm. (Illustration by Lauren Shavell of Medical Imagery.)

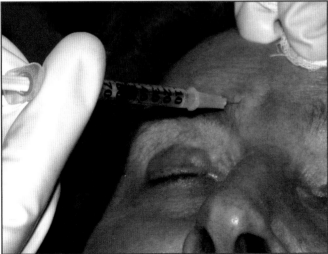

Figure 5-7. Treatment of moderate to severe blepharospasm: In addition to administering a larger dose of BOTOX, the central brow depressors of the glabellum may also require treatment.

Treatment of
Hemifacial Spasm and Meige Syndrome

In contrast to patients with BEB, patients with a history of hemifacial spasm frequently have a history of microvascular disease such as diabetes or hypertension. They may also provide a previous history of trauma that may be associated with aberrant regeneration of the seventh nerve or a history of a previous Bell's palsy with spasticity developing during the recovery period. If the etiology for the condition cannot be determined, it is reasonable to perform a magnetic resonance image (MRI) of the brain and skull base to rule out a space-occupying mass lesion that may impede the function of or irritate the facial nerve along its course. Once an organic cause for hemifacial spasm has been ruled out, treatment with botulinum toxin can be utilized to reduce involuntary contractions of the facial musculature.

Both hemifacial spasm and Meige syndrome are associated with aberrant facial muscle contraction; however, Meige syndrome may also involve the muscles of the neck and induce torticollis. This can be significantly improved by injecting botulinum toxin into the platysma muscles to inactivate their aberrant contraction. Initial starting doses for patients with hemifacial spasm are similar to patients with mild to moderate blepharospasm with the exception that additional injections are typically placed into the muscles of the mid and lower face or neck as indicated. The mid facial muscles that are commonly involved include zygomaticus major and minor, while the platysma is the most commonly involved muscle of the neck. Typically 5 to 10 units of BOTOX are administered to the muscles of the mid face while 10 to 20 units may be used to treat the platysma muscle. Each injection site usually consists of 2.5 to 5 units of BOTOX. If a patient has never received BOTOX injections, it is reasonable to start with 2.5 units per injection site and work up to 5 units to avoid facial asymmetry or depression of the nasolabial fold.

Potential complications for treating the lower face include asymmetry of facial expression, difficulty speaking, and difficulty with chewing or mastication. The injections into the zygomaticus major complex in the mid face should be placed roughly perpendicular to the skin surface. The needle should also be inserted approximately 3 mm to 5 mm below the skin surface to perform a true intramuscular injection. Injections should not be performed below the lateral aspect of the nasal alar cartilage to avoid paralysis of the orbicularis oris muscle that will induce asymmetry of the mouth and lips (Figure 5-8).

Injection of the platysma muscle should be directed at reducing the appearance of the thickened platysmal bands that develop from repeated spastic contraction. Multiple injection sites are employed along the length of the platysmal bands for a total of 2 to 3 injection sites per vertical band with each injection site receiving 2.5 to 5 units of BOTOX (Figure 5-9).

Please see Blepharospasm and Hemifacial Spasm videos on the accompanying DVD.

Figure 5-8. Treatment of hemifacial spasm/Meige syndrome: Typical injection scheme for a patient with hemifacial spasm or Meige syndrome. Injection sites marked with a black "X" indicate regions that would typically receive 5 units of BOTOX while those marked with a gray "O" are regions that may be treated with either 2.5 or 5 units of BOTOX, depending on the frequency and intensity of spasm. (Illustration by Lauren Shavell of Medical Imagery.)

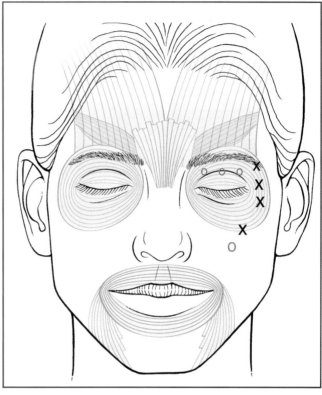

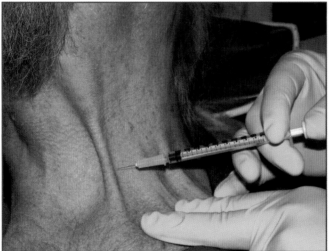

Figure 5-9. Treatment of torticollis and platysmal bands in Meige syndrome: Each injection site consists of 5 units of BOTOX administered along the platysma muscle bands.

References

1. Anderson RL, Patel BC, Holds JB, Jordan DR. Blepharospasm: past, present, and future. *Ophthal Plast Reconstr Surg.* 1998;14(5):305-317.
2. Borodic GE, Cozzolino D. Blepharospasm and its treatment, with emphasis on the use of botulinum toxin. *Plast Reconstr Surg.* 1989;83(3):546-554.
3. Carruthers JD. Ophthalmologic use of botulinum A exotoxin. *Can J Ophthalmol.* 1985;20(4):135-141.
4. Dutton JJ, Buckley EG. Botulinum toxin in the management of blepharospasm. *Arch Neurol.* 1986;43(4):380-382.
5. Frueh BR, Felt DP, Wojno TH, Musch DC. Treatment of blepharospasm with botulinum toxin: a preliminary report. *Arch Ophthalmol.* 1984;102(10):1464-1468.
6. Jankovic J. Botulinum A toxin in the treatment of blepharospasm. *Adv Neurol.* 1988;49:467-472.
7. Jordan DR, Patrinely JR, Anderson RL, Thiese SM. Essential blepharospasm and related dystonias. *Surv Ophthalmol.* 1989;34(2):123-132.
8. McCann JD, Ugurbas SH, Goldberg RA. Benign essential blepharospasm. *Int Ophthalmol Clin.* 2002;42(2):113-121.
9. Biglan AW, May M, Bowers RA. Management of facial spasm with *Clostridium botulinum* toxin, type A (Oculinum). *Arch Otolaryngol Head Neck Surg.* 1988;114(12):1407-1412.
10. Brin MF, Fahn S, Moskowitz C, et al. Localized injections of botulinum toxin for the treatment of focal dystonia and hemifacial spasm. *Mov Disord.* 1987;2(4):237-254.
11. Chen RS, Lu CS, Tsai CH. Botulinum toxin A injection in the treatment of hemifacial spasm. *Acta Neurol Scand.* 1996;94(3):207-211.
12. Evidente VG, Adler CH. Hemifacial spasm and other craniofacial movement disorders. *Mayo Clin Proc.* 1998;73(1):67-71.
13. Mauriello JA, Jr, Leone T, Dhillon S, Pakeman B, Mostafavi R, Yepez MC. Treatment choices of 119 patients with hemifacial spasm over 11 years. *Clin Neurol Neurosurg.* 1996;98(3):213-216.
14. Serrano LA. The use of botulinum toxin type A for the treatment of facial spasm. *Bol Asoc Med P R.* 1993;85(1-3):7-11.
15. Tan EK, Jankovic J. Bilateral hemifacial spasm: a report of five cases and a literature review. *Mov Disord.* 1999;14(2):345-349.
16. Boghen DR, Lesser RL. Blepharospasm and hemifacial spasm. *Curr Treat Options Neurol.* 2000;2(5):393-400.
17. Cuevas C, Madrazo I, Magallon E, Zamorano C, Neri G, Reyes E. Botulinum toxin-A for the treatment of hemifacial spasm. *Arch Med Res.* 1995;26(4):405-408.
18. Defazio G, Abbruzzese G, Girlanda P, et al. Botulinum toxin A treatment for primary hemifacial spasm: a 10-year multicenter study. *Arch Neurol.* 2002;59(3):418-420.
19. Digre K, Corbett JJ. Hemifacial spasm: differential diagnosis, mechanism, and treatment. *Adv Neurol.* 1988;49:151-176.
20. Barker FG 2nd, Jannetta PJ, Bisonette DJ, et al. Microvascular decompression for hemifacial spasm. *J Neurosurg.* 1995;82:201-210.

CHAPTER 6

Treatments for Functional Disorders: Off-Label Uses of Botulinum Toxin

Michael S. McCracken, MD; David B. Granet, MD; and Don O. Kikkawa, MD

Although botulinum toxin has recently gained popularity for cosmetic uses, it was used exclusively for functional indications for many years. Even as cosmetic use becomes increasingly commonplace, more functional uses are rapidly emerging. Presently, there are 2 preparations for botulinum toxin type-A (BOTOX and Dysport) and 1 preparation for botulinum toxin type-B (MYOBLOC). Unless otherwise specified in this chapter, unit doses refer to BOTOX.

Ocular and Periocular Uses

STRABISMUS

In 1973, Scott demonstrated the efficacy and safety of botulinum toxin type-A in weakening the extraocular muscles.[1] He published his clinical results, which demonstrated that botulinum toxin injections are capable of correcting up to 40 prism diopters of deviation 7 years later.[1] The effectiveness of treatment in strabismus is due to the lengthening of an extraocular muscle paralyzed by botulinum toxin type-A and the contraction of its antagonist. Although the effect of botulinum toxin lasts only 5 to 8 weeks when used in extraocular muscles, the temporary changes caused by botulinum toxin type-A may result in lasting improvement in the alignment of eyes. Its uses for strabismus include infantile esotropia, sixth nerve palsy, acquired misalignment in thyroid ophthalmopathy, postsurgical over- and undercorrections, and acquired nystagmus (oscillopsia). More than 200 articles have been published outlining indications and outcomes for botulinum toxin type-A and strabismus since Scott's ground-breaking work.[1-3]

Botulinum toxin type-A has been shown to be effective for the following indications:

* Small-to-moderate–angle esotropia and exotropia
* Postoperative residual strabismus (2 to 8 weeks or more following surgery)

* Weakening of an antagonist muscle in acute paralytic strabismus (especially during sixth nerve palsy)[4,5]

* Cyclic esotropia

* Active thyroid ophthalmopathy (ie, Graves' disease) or inflamed or prephthisical eyes where surgery is inappropriate

In contrast, botulinum toxin type-A has been proven ineffective for the following indications:

* Large-angle deviations (>40 prism D)

* Restrictive or mechanical strabismus (trauma or multiple operations)

* Secondary strabismus due to over-recession of a muscle

* A and V patterns

* Dissociated vertical deviations

* Oblique disorders

* Chronic paralytic strabismus

Multiple treatments are often required for success. In patients undergoing botulinum toxin type-A injections, 72% have maintained a deviation of 10 prism D or less in small-angle esotropia and 33% for large-angle esotropia. Adults and children appear to have similar responses.

Only trained strabismus surgeons should perform these injections. Selected adults can be treated in the clinic setting, while children and more anxious adults require sedation. Although a recent report advocates injection without electromyography,[4] we recommend electromyographic (EMG) guidance. In our experience, guidance is best obtained under topical anesthesia with placement of a unipolar needle into the overacting extraocular muscle during relaxation of the muscle. Electromyography during slow activation of the muscle is then used to ensure proper needle placement. Botulinum toxin injection is most effective when placed at the motor endplate, which is approximately 8 mm posterior to the muscle insertion. The optimal dose typically varies from 1.25 to 5 units per injection. Special 27-gauge, 1.5-inch-long, Teflon-coated, monopolar injection needles are used. The needle is placed in the region of the extraocular muscle. The eye is then turned in the direction that activates the muscle being injected. The toxin is injected once the EMG unit indicates activity. The muscle of the fully sedated patient is injected with direct visualization with or without a conjunctival incision. Side effects and complications may include globe perforation, overcorrection, recurrence of strabismus necessitating repeated injections, and induced vertical diplopia and ptosis.

Botulinum toxin type-A has also been efficacious in treating restrictive strabismus in thyroid-associated orbitopathy.[6,7] This application is especially useful during the phase of active inflammation when surgery is contraindicated. As an isolated procedure, we recommend 10 to 15 units (usual concentration of 5 units/0.1 cc) injected into the center of the belly of the restricted muscle. EMG guidance may be used to confirm intramuscular injection sites. In conjunction with orbital decompression for thyroid orbitopathy, we recommend the injection of 20 units into thickened medial or inferior rectus muscles under direct visualization (Figure 6-1). Although this may cause transient postoperative diplopia due to underaction of the injected extraocular muscle, in our experience it decreases postoperative overaction of thickened extraocular muscles, which may expand into the additional orbital volume created by decompression of the adjacent wall.

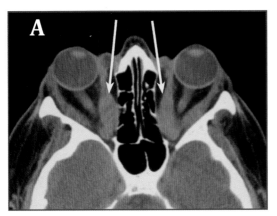 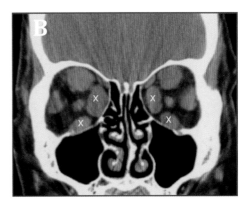

Figure 6-1. Sites for intramuscular injection of BOTOX during orbital decompression: (A) axial and (B) coronal views. X = 10 to 15 units.

Side effects and complications of botulinum toxin injection for strabismus fall into the following 3 categories:

1. Procedural complications: Globe perforation is the most feared complication. Myopia and previous surgery are the main risk factors for this complication. Intravitreal botulinum toxin injection appears to have no toxic effect. Scleral perforations are usually treated successfully with cryotherapy. Retrobulbar and conjunctival hemorrhage and headache are other procedural complications. Retrobulbar hemorrhage requires urgent canthotomy and cantholysis following standard recommendations.

2. Adjacent muscle effects: Ptosis due to levator involvement is the most commonly seen complication, followed by vertical deviations after horizontal rectus injections. Pupillary dilation is a rare side effect caused by ciliary ganglion injection.

3. Sensory effects: Diplopia and spatial disorientation can occur as a result of changing long-standing strabismus patterns (eg, changing an esotropia to an exotropia). These side effects should be discussed preoperatively, as with any strabismus surgery.

TREATMENT OF REFLEX BROW ELEVATION AFTER PTOSIS REPAIR

Frequently, patients with dermatochalasis or ptosis develop a compensatory reflex brow elevation to raise the excess skin or upper lid from the visual axis. Occasionally, this reflex may persist after blepharoplasty or ptosis repair relieves the visual obstruction. This may result in a surprised appearance, apparent overcorrection, and lagophthalmos. In such cases, we have had success using 10 to 20 units to the frontalis muscle (Figure 6-2). Generally, the brows are in a more anatomic position within 1 week. The effect of the toxin dissipates after 3 to 4 months. However, reflex brow elevation rarely recurs once the cycle is broken.

Figure 6-2. Injection sites to treat residual reflex brow elevation after ptosis repair. X = 5 units. (Illustration by Lauren Shavell of Medical Imagery.)

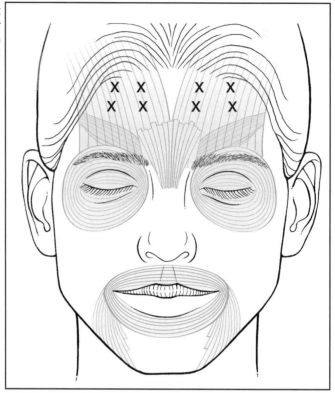

REDUCTION OF GLABELLAR FURROWS IN THYROID-ASSOCIATED ORBITOPATHY

Corrugator overaction, most likely a protective mechanism for eyelid retraction, causes the glabellar rhytides commonly seen in thyroid-related orbitopathy.[8] Olver describes good results treating the corrugator and procerus with 40 units of Dysport[9] (approximately equivalent to 8 to 13 units of BOTOX). We recommend treatment with 25 units shown in Figure 6-3. The effect is seen within 1 week and should last approximately 4 months. One out of 13 patients in Olver's study encountered transient ptosis.[9]

REDUCTION OF UPPER EYELID RETRACTION IN THYROID-ASSOCIATED ORBITOPATHY

Upper eyelid retraction is a common manifestation in patients with thyroid-associated orbitopathy and is traditionally treated by eyelid recession surgery.[10,11] Biglan demonstrated temporary correction by the transcutaneous injection of botulinum toxin type-A between the orbital roof and the levator palpebrae superioris muscle (Figure 6-4).[12] This is best performed with a tuberculin syringe and a 27-gauge needle. Biglan recommended the following doses: 3 units, 5 units, or 7 units for mild, moderate, or severe retraction, respectively.[12] More recently, Traisk and Tallstedt found reduction in eyelid retraction in all 9 patients injected with 2.5 units in a similar fashion.[13] Transcutaneous injections are effective for 6 to 20 weeks.[13] Uddin and Davies have more recently recommended the injection of 2.5 to 7.5 units into the levator and Müller's muscles via the transconjunctival route after the instillation of topical anesthesia.[14]

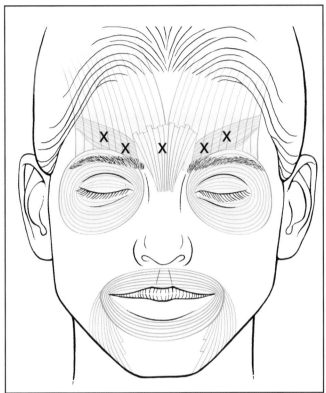

Figure 6-3. Injection sites for glabellar rhytides in thyroid-associated orbitopathy. X = 5 units. (Illustration by Lauren Shavell of Medical Imagery.)

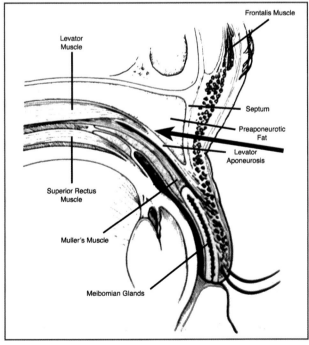

Figure 6-4. Orbital injection site for treatment of upper eyelid retraction in thyroid-associated orbitopathy and for creation of a chemical tarsorrhaphy. See text for dosages. (Adapted from Nerad JA. *Oculoplastic Surgery: The Requisites.* New York: Mosby; 2001.)

Possible complications of toxin injection for upper eyelid retraction in thyroid-associated orbitopathy include ptosis, diplopia, and hypotropia due to binding of toxin at the motor endplates of the superior rectus muscle.

CREATION OF A CHEMICAL TARSORRHAPHY

A suture tarsorrhaphy is traditionally used to protect the cornea in cases of corneal ulceration or to prevent corneal ulceration in patients with fifth and/or seventh nerve palsies. Botulinum toxin type-A may be used to induce a protective ptosis in these cases and has the advantage of allowing easy opening of the lids for instillation of medication or ocular examination without the unreliability of eyelid taping. Botulinum toxin type-A may also be injected in similar fashion in cases of opsoclonus to occlude the affected eye (Figure 6-5). Adams et al reported complete healing of corneal defects in 10 of 13 patients treated with chemical tarsorrhaphy via the transcutaneous route.[15] The toxin is injected in a similar location as described above for treatment of upper lid retraction in thyroid-associated orbitopathy (see Figure 6-4). We recommend 5 to 10 units. After toxin injection, it is crucial to continue taping or medical management until the onset of ptosis, which may take up to 1 week after injection. The effect may last from 3 weeks to 5 months.[15]

The side effects are similar to those listed previously for injection to relieve eyelid retraction in patients with thyroid disease. Persistent hypotropia has been reported after protective ptosis produced by chemical tarsorrhaphy with 7.5 units.[16]

THERAPY OF HYPERLACRIMATION

Gustatory lacrimation ("crocodile tears") describes excessive tearing while eating or smelling food. This syndrome is the result of aberrant regeneration of gustatory nerve fibers, which come to innervate the lacrimal gland. This phenomenon is seen after facial nerve injury due to trauma, surgery, or Bell's palsy. As with blockade of neuromuscular synapses, botulinum toxin has been found to be effective in treating disorders of the autonomic nervous system due to similar blockade of ACh release. Injection of botulinum toxin type-A into the lacrimal gland has been demonstrated to be an effective treatment for gustatory lacrimation.[17-20]

The injection technique is described by Riemann et al.[18] After topical anesthetic drops are instilled in the affected eye, the upper lid is everted to expose the superotemporal bulbar conjunctiva. This is best done under loupe (2.5X) magnification. The transconjunctival approach is then used to gain access to the palpebral lobe of the lacrimal gland with a 30-gauge needle (Figure 6-6). It is critical that the bevel of the needle remain pointed toward the globe to minimize the risk of ocular injury. A 2.5-unit dose of BOTOX is then injected into the palpebral lobe. Transcutaneous injections into the lacrimal gland and orbital orbicularis oculi have been used to treat this condition, but they are associated with a significant risk of ptosis and lagophthalmos.[17,19,20] Therefore, we recommend the transconjunctival route.

The effect is usually apparent several days to 1 week later, and patients are asymptomatic for 3 to 6 months.[17-20] Theoretical side effects include subconjunctival hemorrhage, ptosis, diplopia, and inadvertent penetrating injury of the globe. When treating gustatory epiphora, it is important to rule out other causes of epiphora such as functional lacrimal obstruction and reflex epiphora from exposure keratitis. This is because botulinum toxin treatment will not improve, and may even worsen, these conditions.

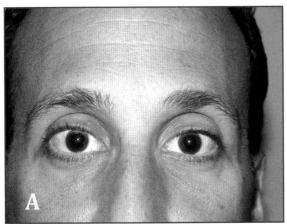

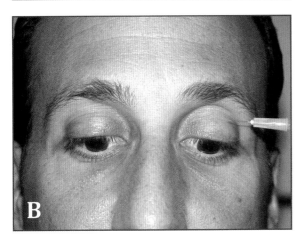

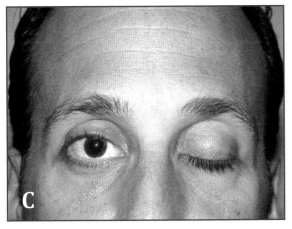

Figure 6-5. Patient with opsoclonus. (A) Before injection. (B) Needle indicates location of injection into levator muscle. (C) Five days after botulinum type-A chemical tarsorrhaphy.

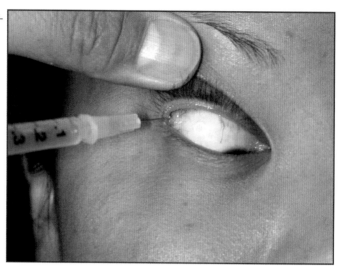

Figure 6-6. Injection site for hyper-lacrimation. Total dose = 2.5 units.

TREATMENT OF DRY EYE

Punctual plugs are commonly used for dry eyes that are not controlled with lubrication, but some patients do not tolerate punctal plugs. Botulinum toxin type-A has been injected into the medial lower lid or the medial upper and lower lids of such patients in order to evert the puncta and decrease tear drainage into the lacrimal sac. One preliminary study of this application has shown promising results.[21] However, further study of this technique is necessary before firm recommendations can be made.

TREATMENT OF SPASTIC LOWER LID ENTROPION

Some patients with spastic lower lid entropion may be poor surgical candidates or be unwilling to undergo surgical repair. The mechanism of relief is due to orbicularis paralysis, which eliminates one of the contributing anatomical conditions responsible for entropion. Interestingly, the effect of botulinum toxin treatment for entropion is simulated by the immediate resolution of entropion immediately after the injection of local anesthetic in patients undergoing standard entropion repair. In such patients, temporary relief may be obtained by the injection of 10 to 15 units of BOTOX into the preseptal orbicularis muscle of the lower lid (Figure 6-7).[22-24] Such injection will result in correction of entropion that may last as long as 3 to 4 months, but entropion usually recurs without repeated injection. Complications for patients treated with botulinum toxin for lower lid entropion include paralytic ectropion (overcorrection), epiphora due to punctal eversion, and diplopia due to inferior oblique weakening.

TREATMENT OF GUSTATORY EPIPHORA

Gustatory epiphora or "crocodile tears" is a condition characterized by excessive lacrimation while eating or smelling food. It usually occurs after a seventh nerve palsy (eg, Bell's palsy, stroke) and is thought to be due to misdirected or aberrant regeneration of salivary nerve fibers directed to the lacrimal gland. As with blockade of neuromuscular synapses, botulinum toxin has been found to be effective in disorders of the autonomic nervous system due to similar blockade of ACh release. Boroojerdi et al were the first to demonstrate the improvement in gustatory epiphora with the injection of botulinum

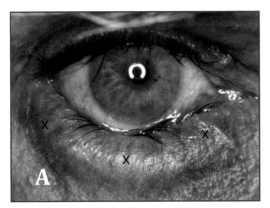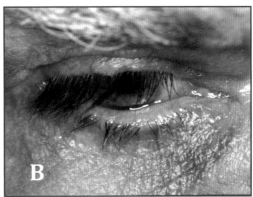

Figure 6-7. Lower lid entropion (A) before and (B) after injection of botulinum toxin type A. X = 5 units.

toxin into the lacrimal gland.[17] Other studies have corroborated their results.[17,18,20] Both BOTOX (2.5 to 5 units) and Dysport (average of 20 units) have been used.[19,20]

Mild eyelid synkinesis also occurs in patients with aberrant seventh nerve regeneration. This condition can be treated in a manner similar to essential blepharospasm and hemifacial spasm. When treating gustatory epiphora, it is important to rule out other causes of epiphora such as functional lacrimal obstruction and reflex epiphora from exposure keratitis. This is because botulinum toxin treatment will not improve, and may even worsen, these conditions.

Two routes of injection have been described: transcutaneous and transconjunctival. Riemann et al reported the use of 2.5 units of BOTOX (diluted in 100 units per 5 mL of solution) into the palpebral lobe of the lacrimal gland between the secretory orifices under an everted upper lid.[18]

Hofmann injected 5 units of BOTOX (diluted in 100 units per 3 mL of solution) into the lacrimal gland through the transcutaneous route just beneath the orbital rim.[25] Other studies used an average of 20 units of Dysport through the transcutaneous route.[19]

Botulinum toxin treatment is contraindicated in patients in whom epiphora is not a true hyperlacrimation. This includes patients with a seventh nerve palsy with epiphora due to functional obstruction or reflex epiphora (eg, exposure keratitis). The development of dry eye is a theoretical risk of treatment, but this was not reported in the studies cited. Ptosis and superior rectus underaction were reported in 1 patient undergoing a transcutaneous botulinum toxin injection,[18] and pre-existing ptosis worsened in another.[19]

TREATMENT OF APRAXIA OF EYELID OPENING

Apraxia of lid opening is the inability to initiate eyelid opening (Figure 6-8). It may be noted in patients suffering from blepharospasm. It is felt to be due to pretarsal orbicularis oculi activity, which is not evident on clinical examination.[26-28] Forget et al demonstrated an improvement in eyelid opening after the injection of 4 to 5 units into 4 sites.[29] We typically inject 2 sites per upper eyelid (Figure 6-9).

AS AN ADJUNCT TO FACIAL WOUND HEALING

Preoperative planning allows incision placement along the relaxed skin tension lines to allow minimization of tension on the wounds. In some situations, such as trauma, wounds are not parallel to the relaxed skin tension lines. In such cases, measures must

Figure 6-8. Patient with apraxia of eyelid opening, shown during attempted eyelid opening.

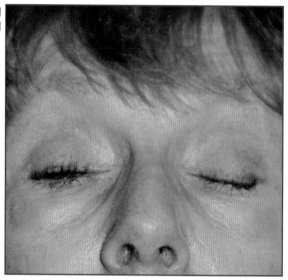

Figure 6-9. Injection sites for treatment of apraxia of eyelid opening. X = 5 units. (Illustration by Lauren Shavell of Medical Imagery.)

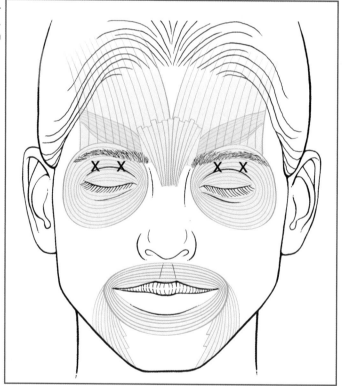

be taken to minimize tension on the incision in order to ensure optimum wound healing. These measures traditionally include deep layer closure and skin undermining. Sherris and Gassner reported the use of botulinum toxin type-A to minimize tension during the healing of a 15-mm laceration of the supraorbital rim.[30] In this report, the frontalis muscle was injected with 10 units and the ipsilateral corrugator and frontalis were injected with a total of 7.5 units. A 2-layered closure was also utilized. Of note, the authors advocate

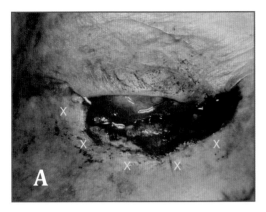
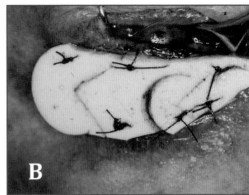
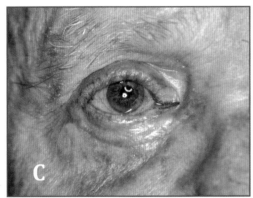

Figure 6-10. Patient with reconstructed lower eyelid. (A) Intraoperative defect with injection sites. (B) Reconstructed lid, after placement of bolster. (C) Postoperative result after resolution of toxin effect. X = 5 units.

reconstitution of the toxin with lidocaine 1% with 1:100,000 epinephrine.[30,31] The rapid onset of action of the lidocaine allows the physician to confirm that the botulinum toxin type-A injection is appropriately placed to paralyze the muscles that will cause wound tension.

Choi et al[32] demonstrated the effectiveness of botulinum toxin type-A in immobilization of reconstructed eyelids. We have found this application particularly useful. We show a sample injection pattern (Figure 6-10A) used during reconstruction of a lower lid with a bolster for additional immobilization during the first postoperative week (Figure 6-10B). This patient had excellent postoperative results (Figure 6-10C).

Applications in Therapy of Hyperhidrosis

Botulinum toxin type-A has been shown to reduce localized sweat production by inhibiting the cholinergic innervation of the eccrine and apocrine sweat glands.[33]

Axillary Hyperhidrosis

Randomized, double-blinded studies have demonstrated the efficacy of botulinum toxin type-A injections in treating axillary hyperhidrosis.[34-36]

Minor's iodine-starch test may be used to mark the extent of the area to be injected, but we feel this is not necessary to achieve satisfactory results. Although doses ranging from 15 units[37] to 200 units per axilla[38,39] have been administered, a total dose of 50 units per axilla provides a reliable response without the theoretical risk of development of antibodies to the toxin. Naver et al reported a median duration of 9 months of effect after the axillary injection of 38 to 72 units.[40] Karamfilov et al and Wollina et al recommend higher doses for a longer effect and reported a 16.7% relapse rate at up to 15 months follow-up[38] and a 12.8% relapse rate at up to 29 months follow-up,[39] respectively. The toxin should be injected intradermally with a 30-gauge needle, and it is distributed over 10 to 20 sites per axilla.

The effect may be noticed as soon as 3 days after injection.[41,42] It is usually noticed within a week and may last from several months to 29 months.[39] Higher doses may provide a longer duration of effect.[38,39] Interestingly, axillary injections have been demonstrated to improve body odor.[43]

Side effects of axillary injections may include localized hematomas. At least 1 patient has reported ulnar paresthesias after such injection.[44] We are unaware of muscle weakness or the development of antibodies to botulinum toxin type-A after axillary injection.

Of note, botulinum toxin type-B has also been shown to be effective in axillary hyperhidrosis at a dose of 2000 units per axilla.[45]

The effectiveness of these injections should not be trivialized because they have shown that they improve the quality of life in patients with axillary hyperhidrosis who often suffer from multiple emotional and social impairments.[46,47]

PALMAR HYPERHIDROSIS

Botulinum toxin type-A has also demonstrated efficacy in the treatment of palmar hyperhidrosis.[48-52] Median and ulnar nerve blocks, as well as brachial plexus blocks, have been performed to provide anesthesia for palmar injections.[53,54] However, such blocks cause a transient palsy. Furthermore, they have a rare incidence of neurologic damage, particularly when they are repeated over time.[55] Alternative methods of anesthesia include topical anesthesia, ice pack application,[56] and monitored anesthesia care with intravenous propofol.

As with axillary injections, Minor's iodine-starch test may be used to identify the area of hyperhidrosis. If this test is utilized, a marking pen can then be used to divide the hyperhidrotic area into squares measuring 20 cm by 20 cm. Each square can then serve as an injection site.[57] Alternatively, the injections may be placed into the palms at sites that are a given distance apart. This distance may range from 10 mm to 25 mm.[40,41,53,56,54] Saadia et al suggested varying the spacing of injection sites from 15 mm to 25 mm based upon the local response to the Minor's iodine-starch test, with the most hyperhidrotic areas receiving the greater density of injections.[56] Injection into the fingertips may be omitted in an attempt to avoid loss of friction in gripping.[58]

Doses ranging from 28 to 200 units per hand have been advocated.[41,53,54,56] BOTOX may be diluted to yield injections of 1 to 4 units per site,[53,56] with the volume injected per site usually about 0.1 cc. Also, Dysport has been injected successfully at doses ranging from 120 to 250 units per palm.[48,51,52,59]

The injections should be distributed over 16 to 40 sites.[40,53,60] The number of sites may be adjusted according to the size of the patient's hands.[56,60] The injections should be at the intradermal level and may be administered with a 30-gauge needle. Improvement in hyperhidrosis after administration of BOTOX can be expected within 1 week of injection and may last anywhere from 4 to 22 months.[53,54] Side effects of palmar injection include pain on injection, hematoma, muscle weakness, and paresthesias.[40,41,56]

OTHER USES

Diabetic gustatory sweating is marked by localized facial hyperhidrosis during meals. It is felt to be the result of parasympathetic reinnervation of the sweat glands after sympathetic neuropathy.[57,60] Botulinum toxin type-A injections have shown favorable results in treating hyperhidrosis in patients with diabetic gustatory sweating.[61]

Botulinum toxin type-A has proven effective in treating hyperhidrosis in patients with Ross syndrome, which is composed of tonic pupils, areflexia, and localized hyperhidrosis.[62] Botulinum toxin type-A has also shown promise in the treatment of dermatologic conditions exacerbated by moisture, such as dyshidrotic hand eczema,[63] Hailey-Hailey disease (familial benign pemphigus),[64,65] and lichen simplex.[66]

Summary

Adjunct, off-label uses of botulinum toxin type-A continue to be elucidated. We have attempted to highlight a few of these, but we expect many more to be discovered in the years to come.

References

1. Scott AB, Rosenbaum A, Collins C. Pharmacological weakening of extra-ocular muscles. *Invest Ophthalmol Vis Sci.* 1973;12:924-927.
2. McNeer KW, Spencer RF, Tucker MG. Botulinum toxin therapy for essential infantile esotropia in children. *Arch Ophthalmol.* 1997;116:701-702.
3. Benabent EC, Hermosa PG, Arrazola MT, Alio y Sanz JL. Botulinum toxin injection without electromyographic assistance. *J Pediatr Ophthalmol Strabismus.* 2002;39:231-234.
4. Kao LY, Chao AN. Subtenon injection of botulinum toxin for treatment of traumatic sixth nerve palsy. *J Pediatr Ophthalmol Strabismus.* 2003;40:27-30.
5. Holmes JM, Beck RW, Kip KE, et al. Botulinum toxin treatment versus conservative management in acute traumatic sixth nerve palsy or paresis. *J AAPOS.* 2000;4(3):145-149.
6. Dunn WJ, Arnold AC, O'Connor PS. Botulinum toxin for the treatment of dysthyroid ocular myopathy. *Ophthalmology.* 1986;93:470-475.
7. Lyons CJ, Vickers SF, Lee JP. Botulinum toxin therapy in dysthyroid strabismus. *Eye.* 1990;4:538-540.
8. Saks ND, Burnstine MA, Putterman AM. Glabellar rhytides in thyroid-associated orbitopathy. *Ophthal Plast Reconstr Surg.* 2001;17(2):91-95.
9. Olver JM. Botulinum toxin type-A treatment of overactive corrugator supercilii in thyroid eye disease. *Br J Ophthalmol.* 1998;82:528-533.
10. Hedin A. Eyelid surgery in dysthyroid orbitopathy. *Eye.* 1988;2:201-206.
11. Gorve AS. Upper eyelid retraction and Grave's disease. *Ophthalmology.* 1981;88:499-506.
12. Biglan AW. Control of eyelid retraction associated with Graves' disease with botulinum A toxin. *Ophthal Surg.* 1994;25(3):186-188.
13. Traisk F, Tallstedt L. Thyroid-associated ophthalmopathy: botulinum toxin type-A in the treatment of upper eyelid retraction: a pilot study. *Acta Ophthalmol Scand.* 2001;79:585-588.
14. Uddin JM, Davies PD. Treatment of upper eyelid retraction associated with thyroid eye disease with subconjunctival botulinum toxin injection. *Ophthalmology.* 2002;109(6):1183-1187.
15. Adams GG, Kirkness CM, Lee FP. Botulinum toxin type-A induced protective ptosis. *Eye.* 1987;1(Part 5):603-608.
16. Heyworth PLO, Lee FP. Persisting hypotropias following protective ptosis induced by botulinum neurotoxin. *Eye.* 1994;8:511-515.

17. Boroojerdi B, Ferbert A, Schwarz M, et al. Botulinum toxin treatment of synkinesia and hyperlacrimation after facial palsy. *J Neurol Neurosurg Psychiatry.* 1998;65:111-114.

18. Riemann R, Pfennigsdorf S, Riemann E, Naumann M. Successful treatment of crocodile tears by injection of botulinum toxin into the lacrimal gland: a case report. *Ophthalmology.* 1999;106:2322-2324.

19. Montoya FJ, Riddell CE, Caesar R, Hague S. Treatment of gustatory hyperlacrimation (crocodile tears) with injection of botulinum toxin into the lacrimal gland. *Eye.* 2002;16:705-709.

20. Keegan DJ, Geerling G, Lee JP, et al. Botulinum toxin treatment for hyperlacrimation secondary to aberrant regenerated seventh nerve palsy or salivary gland transplantation. *Br J Ophthalmol.* 2002;86:43-46.

21. Sahlin S, Chen E, Kaugesaar T, et al. Effect of eyelid botulinum toxin injection on lacrimal drainage. *Am J Ophthalmol.* 2000;129:481-486.

22. Carruthers J. Ophthalmic use of botulinum A exotoxin. *Can J Ophthalmol.* 1985;20:135-141.

23. Carruthers J, Stubbs HA. Botulinum toxin for benign essential blepharospasm, hemifacial spasm and age-related lower eyelid entropion. *Can J Neurol Sci.* 1987;14:42-45.

24. Clarke JR, Spalton DJ. Treatment of senile entropion with botulinum toxin. *Br J Ophthalmol.* 1988;72:361-362.

25. Hofmann RJ. Treatment of Frey's syndrome (gustatory sweating) and "crocodile tears" (gustatory epiphora) with purified botulinum toxin. *Ophthal Plast Reconstr Surg.* 2000;16:289-291.

26. Elston JS. A new variant of blepharospasm. *J Neurol Neurosurg Psychiatry.* 1992;55:369-371.

27. Aramideh M, Ongerboer de Visser BW, Devriese PP, et al. Electromyographic features of levator palpebrae superioris and orbicularis oculi muscles in blepharospasm. *Brain.* 1994;117:27-38.

28. Tozlovanu V, Forget R, Iancu A, Boghen D. Prolonged orbicularis oculi activity: a major factor in apraxia of lid opening. *Neurology.* 2001;57:1013-1018.

29. Forget R, Tozlovanu V, Iancu A, Boghen D. Botulinum toxin improves lid opening delays in blepharospasm-associated apraxia of lid opening. *Neurology.* 2002;58:1843-1846.

30. Sherris DA, Gassner HG. Botulinum toxin to minimize facial scarring. *Facial Plast Surg.* 2002;18(1):35-39.

31. Gassner HG, Sherris DA. Addition of anesthetic agent enhances the predictability of botulinum toxin injections. *Mayo Clin Proc.* 2000;75:701-704.

32. Choi JC, Lucarelli MJ, Shore JW. Use of botulinum A toxin in patients at risk of wound complications following eyelid reconstruction. *Ophthal Plast Reconstr Surg.* 1997;13(4):259-264.

33. Heckmann M, Schaller M, Ceballos-Baumann A, Plewig M. Follow-up of patients with axillary hyperhidrosis after botulinum toxin injection. *Arch Dermatol.* 1998;134(10):1298-1299.

34. Schnider P, Binder M, Kittler H, et al. A randomized, double-blind, placebo-controlled trial of botulinum A toxin for severe axillary hyperhidrosis. *Br J Dermatol.* 1999;140(4):677-680.

35. Heckmann M, Ceballos-Baumann A, Plewig G, for the Hyperhidrosis Study Group. Botulinum toxin type-A for axillary hyperhidrosis (excessive sweating). *N Engl J Med.* 2001;344(7):488-493.

36. Naumann M, Lowe NJ, on behalf of the Hyperhidrosis Clinical Study Group. Botulinum toxin type-A in treatment of bilateral primary axillary hyperhidrosis: randomized, parallel group, double blind, placebo controlled trial. *BMJ.* 2001;323:596-599.

37. Bushara KO, Park DM, Jones JC, Schutta HS. Botulinum toxin: a possible new treatment for axillary hyperhidrosis. *Clin Exp Dermatol.* 1996;21:276-278.

38. Karamfilov T, Konrad H, Karte K, Wollina U. Lower relapse rate of botulinum toxin type-A therapy for axillary hyperhidrosis by dose increase. *Arch Dermatol.* 2000;136:487-490.

39. Wollina U, Karamfilov T, Konrad H. High-dose botulinum toxin type-A therapy for axillary hyperhidrosis markedly prolongs the relapse-free interval. *J Am Acad Dermatol.* 2002;46(4):536-540.

40. Naver H, Swartling C, Aquilonius SM. Palmar and axillary hyperhidrosis treated with botulinum toxin: one-year clinical follow-up. *Eur J Neurology.* 2000;7(1):55-62.

41. Naumann M, Hofmann U, Bergmann I, et al. Focal hyperhidrosis: effective treatment with intracutaneous botulinum toxin. *Arch Dermatol.* 1998;134(3):301-304.

42. Akdeniz S, Harman M, Aluclu U, Alp S. Axillary hyperhidrosis treated with botulinum toxin type-A exotoxin. *J Eur Acad Dermatol Venereol.* 2002;16(2):171-172.

43. Heckmann M, Teichmann B, Pause B, Plewig G. Amelioration of body odor after intracutaneous axillary injection of botulinum toxin type-A. *Arch Dermatol.* 2003;139:57-59.

44. Naumann M, Bergmann I, Hofmann U, et al. Botulinum toxin for focal hyperhidrosis: technical considerations and improvements in application. *Br J Derm.* 1998;139(6):1123-1124.
45. Dressler D, Saberi F, Benecke R. Botulinum toxin type-B for treatment of axillary hyperhidrosis. *J Neurol.* 2002;249:1729-1732.
46. Swartling C, Naer H, Lindberg M. Botulinum A toxin improves life quality in severe primary focal hyperhidrosis. *Eur J Neurol.* 2001;8:247-252.
47. Tan SR, Solish N. Long-term efficacy and quality of life in the treatment of focal hyperhidrosis with botulinum toxin type-A. *Derm Surg.* 2002;28(6):495-499.
48. Schnider P, Binder M, Auff E, et al. Double-blind trial of botulinum A toxin for the treatment of focal hyperhidrosis of the palms. *Br J Dermatol.* 1997;136:548-552.
49. Shelley WB, Talanin NY, Shelley ED. Botulinum toxin therapy for palmar hyperhidrosis. *J Am Acad Dermatol.* 1998;38:227-229.
50. Holmes S, Mann C. Botulinum toxin in the treatment of palmar hyperhidrosis. *J Am Acad Dermatol.* 1998;39:1040-1041.
51. Heckmann M, Scaller M, Plewig G, Ceballos-Baumann A. Optimizing botulinum toxin therapy for hyperhidrosis. *Br J Dermatol.* 1998;138:553-554.
52. Naver H, Aquilonius SM. The treatment of focal hyperhidrosis with botulinum toxin. *Arch Dermatol.* 1998;134:301-304.
53. Vadoud-Seyedi J, Heenen M, Simonart T. Treatment of idiopathic palmar hyperhidrosis with botulinum toxin: report of 23 cases and review of the literature. *Dermatology.* 2001;203:318-321.
54. Wollina U, Karamfilov T. Botulinum toxin type-A for palmar hyperhidrosis. *J Eur Acad Dermatol Venereol.* 2001;15:555-558.
55. Hernot S, Samii K. Different types of nerve injuries in locoregional anesthesia. *Ann Fr Anesth Reanim.* 1997;16:923-924.
56. Saadia D, Voustianiouk A, Wang AK, Kaufmann H. Botulinum toxin type-A in primary palmar hyperhidrosis: randomized, single-blind, two-dose study. *Neurology.* 2001;57:2095-2099.
57. Paparella MM, Shumrick DA. Complications of parotid gland surgery. *Otolaryngology.* 1991;104:2117-2127.
58. Schnider P, Moraru E, Kittler H, et al. Treatment of focal hyperhidrosis with botulinum toxin type A: long-term follow-up in 61 patients. *Br J Dermatol.* 2001;145:289-293.
59. Goldman A. Treatment of axillary and palmar hyperhidrosis with botulinum toxin. *Aesth Plast Surg.* 2000;24:280-282.
60. Kurchin A, Adar R, Zweig A, Mozes M. Gustatory phenomena after upper dorsal sympathectomy. *Arch Neurol.* 1977;34:619-623.
61. Restivo DA, Lanza S, Patti F, et al. Improvement of diabetic autonomic gustatory sweating by botulinum toxin type A. *Neurology.* 2002;59:1971-1973.
62. Bergmann I, Dauphin M, Naumann M, et al. Selective degeneration of sudomotor fibers in Ross syndrome and successful treatment of compensatory hyperhidrosis with botulinum toxin. *Muscle Nerve.* 1998;21:1790-1793.
63. Wollina U, Karamfilov T. Adjuvant botulinum toxin type-A in dyshidrotic hand eczema: a controlled prospective pilot study with left-right comparison. *J Eur Acad Dermatol Venereol.* 2002;16:40-42.
64. Lapiere JC, Hirsh A, Gordon KB, et al. Botulinum toxin type-A for the treatment of axillary Hailey-Hailey disease. *Dermatol Surg.* 2000;26:371-374.
65. Kang N, Yoon T, Kim T. Botulinum toxin type-A as an effective adjuvant therapy for Hailey-Hailey disease. *Dermatol Surg.* 2002;28(6):543-544.
66. Heckmann M, Heyer G, Brunner B, Plewig G. Botulinum toxin type-A injection in the treatment of lichen simplex: an open pilot study. *J Am Acad Dermatol.* 2002;46(4):617-619.

Financial disclosure: Dr. Granet is a consultant for Alcon, Insite Vision, and Diopsys, Inc.

CHAPTER 7

Botulinum Toxin as a Treatment for Headache

Patrick K. Johnson, MD and William J. Lipham, MD, FACS

Headaches are not only painful and disabling for patients but also incur a huge economic burden on society. Chronic headaches affect over 45 million Americans, over half of whom have migraine headaches.[1] There is a direct medical cost of over $9.5 billion/year, with indirect costs as high as $13 billion/year due to decreased productivity, since headaches are felt to cause workers to miss more than 112 million days from work annually.[2] Headaches are also a common cause for emergency room admissions. The costs of such visits have been reported to be between $717 million and $2.15 billion.[3,4]

The 4 major types of headaches include migraine, tension-type headache (TTH), chronic daily headache (CDH), and cluster headache. Until recently, treatment of these disorders has been primarily abortive in nature and in the case of migraine, extremely expensive. This has spurred interest to pursue potential prophylactic measures to decrease both the frequency and intensity of all forms of headache. A serendipitous observation by Dr. William Binder, an ears, nose, and throat (ENT) surgeon, in 1992 led to the study of botulinum toxin use in the treatment of headache. Dr. Binder noted that many of his patients who had been treated with botulinum toxin for hyperfunctional glabellar lines reported a significant reduction or complete elimination of their migraine headaches. His initial findings suggest that botulinum toxin may play a preventive role in the treatment of migraine headache. This has led to a number of clinical trials to determine the utility of botulinum toxin type-A in the treatment of not only migraine headache, but also TTH and CDH.[5] The focus of this chapter will be to provide readers with the diagnostic criteria, pathophysiology, current treatment regimen, and finally the role of botulinum toxin in the treatment for each of these headache varieties.

Background and Epidemiology

Migraine is a common and disabling disorder affecting 18% of women and 6% of men. The incidence of migraine is as high as 35% in women at age 40.[1] Migraines are 3 times more common in women than in men and migraines often run in families. A typical patient is an otherwise healthy young woman. Migraine differs from TTH in that migraine is usually associated with vegetative symptoms, including nausea, photophobia, and phonophobia. They are unilateral in 60% to 70% of cases and are usually gradual in onset with a crescendo pattern. Migraines are usually pulsating with moderate or severe intensity and are often aggravated by routine physical activity.[6,7] Since migraine headaches are frequently debilitating, they have a significant socioeconomic impact due to loss of productivity because many patients are frequently bed-ridden and unable to work.

There are 3 different types of migraine headaches: migraine with aura, migraine without aura, and migraine variants. Aura occurs in less than 20% of migraine sufferers. While a variety of medications have been used for the preventive treatment of migraine, only 5 have been FDA approved for the treatment of migraine: propranolol, timolol, divalproex sodium, methysergide, and topiramate. The search for a better tolerated and more effective migraine preventive agent continues in earnest.

TTH, although usually much less disabling than migraine, is far more common, with a lifetime prevalence of 61%.[1] Like migraine headaches, tension headaches are more prevalent in women but to a lesser extent (female:male ratio is approximately 1.5:1). The typical age of onset is around age 20 and prevalence is felt to decline with age.[8] Tension headaches tend to be bilateral and have a feeling of pressure or tightness, frequently in a hat-band distribution that waxes or wanes in severity.[9]

CDH is defined as having more than 15 days of headache per month.[10] The 2 most common subtypes are chronic TTH and chronic migraine. While patients with CDH often have underlying migraine, the headache pattern is more typical of TTH. CDH affects about 3% to 5% of the population or approximately 8.1 to 13.5 million individuals in the United States.[11,12] More than 90% of patients start with episodic headaches or migraines and progress to CDH. Abortive attempts to treat the pain with analgesic overuse is often associated with this evolution.[13,14]

Cluster headaches are less prevalent than migraine, TTH, or CDH with a prevalence of about 0.1%.[15] Cluster headaches, unlike the other types of headaches, typically affect more men than women at a ratio of approximately 5:1. Cluster headaches are always unilateral and most often begin around the eye or temple. Pain begins quickly and reaches its most severe point in minutes. The pain is deep and excruciating.[16]

The International Headache Society has established diagnostic criteria for migraines and other headaches. Currently, once a diagnosis has been made, a wide variety of abortive treatments are available, but the efficacy and cost of those treatments may not be desirable. There is a broad array of studies underway to determine if botulinum toxin type-A may serve a role in decreasing the frequency and severity of a variety of headaches, including those previously described. Researchers are hopeful that this treatment may decrease the dependency on abortive medications that play a role in the management of headache but are frequently inadequate and expensive.

Pathophysiology

There are 4 pathophysiologic hypotheses concerning the development of migraine headache.[17,18] These include the vascular theory, the cortical spreading depression (CSD) hypothesis, the neurovascular hypothesis, and the serotonergic abnormality hypothesis.

The vascular theory suggests that migraine is a vasospastic disorder that begins with vasoconstriction in the cranial vasculature (aura) and is followed by dilation of the intracranial or extracranial blood vessels.

The CSD hypothesis suggests that migraines begin with a period of neuronal excitation, followed by a much longer period of neuronal depression, which causes disturbances in neuronal metabolism and a reduction in blood flow, which is felt to be involved in the aura phase of a migraine.

The neurovascular hypothesis suggests that either migraine triggers or CSD can activate trigeminal nerve axons, which release neuropeptides (substance P, calcitonin gene-related peptide [CGRP], and neurokinin A) from axon terminals near the meningeal and other blood vessels. CGRP is a potent vasodilator and substance P and neurokinin A also cause vasodilatation and will promote extravasation of plasma proteins and fluid from the meningeal blood vessels. This causes an inflammatory response around the innervated blood vessels.

The serotonergic abnormality hypothesis suggests that a dysfunction in serotonin levels may also cause migraine headaches. When platelets become activated, they release serotonin and increase the plasma serotonin level. An increase in serotonin level causes vasoconstriction; likewise a drop in serotonin causes vasodilation. Platelet serotonin levels drop and vasodilation occurs during a migraine attack. This suggests that there is an increase in serotonin release during a migraine attack. This initial surge of serotonin is thought to cause the aura phase. The subsequent drop in serotonin levels, causing vasodilation of the blood vessels, is thought to cause the headache phase.

The classical theory of TTH (ie, muscle contraction in the head and neck produces vasoconstriction and ischemia) is no longer in favor.[19] One theory of TTH is the concept of a headache continuum. In this theory, TTHs are mild to moderate at one end of the spectrum and migraines are at the moderate to severe end of the spectrum.[20] Another theory suggests that a trigeminal neurovascular system and unstable serotonergic neurotransmission may play a role in TTH.[21]

Cluster headaches and the underlying pathophysiology remain unclear. It is thought that the basic pathophysiology is in the hypothalamic gray matter.[22] While vasodilation does occur and may be responsible for the pain and autonomic features of the cluster headache, it is most likely extracerebral and seems to be secondary to neuronal dysfunction.[23,24]

Current Therapies

PHARMACOLOGICAL TREATMENT OF MIGRAINE

Pharmaceuticals have been used to both treat and prevent migraine headaches. Abortive therapy usually starts prior to coming to the physician's office with over-the-counter medication such as a nonsteroidal anti-inflammatory drug (NSAID) or acetaminophen.

There are many migraine-specific agents for migraine therapy. Seven serotonin 1b/1d agonists (triptans) are available for oral, subcutaneous, and intranasal administration. Triptans are most effective when used early in the migraine and promote vasoconstriction in the brain.[25] Ergotamine and dihydroergotamine can also be used for abortive therapy. Dihydroergotamine, available in intravenous, intramuscular, and intranasal forms, offers a more favorable side effect profile to ergotamine and is used often when patients have passed the time frame in which the triptans would be beneficial or if the patient is subject to headache recurrence or rebound.[26]

PHARMACOLOGICAL TREATMENT OF TENSION HEADACHE

Treatment of TTH usually starts with simple analgesics such as acetaminophen, aspirin, or other NSAIDs. When the headaches become chronic, tricyclic antidepressants are commonly used for prophylaxis.

PHARMACOLOGICAL TREATMENT OF CHRONIC DAILY HEADACHE

The outpatient treatment of CDH may be challenging because the headache may be caused by overuse of abortive pain-relief medications. Medication overuse can obscure the diagnosis of CDH and a 2-month period of cessation of medication overuse is required to establish the diagnosis of CDH with certainty.

PHARMACOLOGICAL TREATMENT OF CLUSTER HEADACHE

Cluster headache is harder to treat due to the short time frame of each episode; however, there are therapeutic options. Inhaling 6 L/min of oxygen by a nonrebreathing mask for 15 minutes has been shown to abort cluster headaches.[27] Sumatriptan administered subcutaneously has been shown to decrease the severity of the headache by 74% 15 minutes after treatment, and 36% of patients were completely pain free 10 minutes after administration.[28] Intranasal sumatriptan has been found effective, although the speed of response is slower than what is seen with the subcutaneous injections.

The Role of Botulinum Toxin Type-A for the Treatment of Headache

Over the last few years there has been continually emerging evidence for the role of botulinum toxin type-A in the treatment of migraine headaches, tension headaches, and CDH. The exact mechanism as to why botulinum toxin type-A is effective in reducing the frequency and severity of migraine, TTH, or CDH is not clear. It is well known that the toxin causes muscle paralysis by blocking ACh release at the neuromuscular junction.

A great deal of skepticism was generated as initial case reports and open label series were reported. Controversy stemmed from the inability to reconcile the major mechanism of action of botulinum toxin (blockade of the neuromuscular junction) with concepts of migraine as a disorder affecting neurons and vascular structures. Skepticism also flourished because initial studies showed greater efficacy of botulinum toxin type-A therapy in migraine headache than in TTH. Recent theories suggest that botulinum toxin is taken up by the nerve terminals of the trigeminal nerves where it not only blocks the release of ACh for neuromuscular transmission but also blocks the release of nociceptive neuropeptides involved in the chronic inflammatory pain response, such as substance P and glutamate. This theoretically inhibits both peripheral and central sensitization, thereby down regulating pain.

In addition, it has been recently demonstrated that botulinum toxin type-A is capable of reducing the release of CGRP from trigeminal nerve cells into the central nervous system.[17] Botulinum toxin type-A may apparently be capable of blocking the release of nociceptive neuropeptides into the brain, which could affect vasodilation and the genesis of migraine headaches.[17]

Botulinum Toxin Type-A in the Treatment of Migraine Headache

Many studies have shown that BOTOX can play a role in the treatment of migraines. Binder et al's initial open-label study reported 96 patients with chronic migraine identified through cosmetic surgery and movement disorder clinics.[5] All patients received injections into the glabellar, temporalis, and occipitalis regions with a mean dose of 26 units. Fifty-one percent of these patients reported complete resolution of headaches, 28% noted greater than 50% improvement in either frequency or severity, and 21% reported no significant response. The average duration of benefit was 3.6 months.

A recent small, blinded, placebo-controlled study enrolled 30 patients with episodic migraine.[29] Patients were treated with a total of 50 units at 6 fixed sites, which included the frontalis, corrugators, procerus, temporalis, splenius capitus, and cervicalis. A greater than 50% reduction in migraine episodes and significant reductions in both headache severity and need for acute medication were demonstrated. More recently, investigators at the Mayo Clinic in Scottsdale, Ariz looked at reduction in disability in a prospective open-label study.[30] Patients with migraine were treated with 25 to 100 units and evaluated using the MIDAS disability scale as the primary outcome. Of these patients, 58% reported a decrease in disability and a full 40% reported an excellent response (>75% improvement).

A number of other studies, mostly open-label and small in size, show promising results of botulinum toxin type-A therapy in headache patients. Allergan (the manufacturer of BOTOX) is currently running several large studies that examine both a fixed-dose protocol and a "follow the pain" protocol. The latter enables the injector to customize the amount of toxin to be injected and the injection sites based on the characteristics of the patient's headaches and the findings on examination, such as the presence of multiple trigger points in the neck.

Botulinum Toxin Type-A in the Treatment of Tension Headache

Patients with cervicogenic headaches and post-traumatic headaches often have daily debilitating headaches that are best characterized as chronic TTH. Smuts et al reported the first double-blind, placebo-controlled study of botulinum toxin type-A in patients with chronic TTH.[31] In this study, 22 patients received botulinum toxin type-A and 15 received placebo. Smuts et al treated the temporalis, the splenius, and the trapezius bilaterally with a total of 100 units. Fifty-nine percent of these patients reported improvement while only 13% of placebo-treated patients noted benefit.

Not all studies, however, show uniformly positive results. Studies by Schulte-Mattler et al and Padberg et al showed no statistical significance.[32,33]

Botulinum Toxin Type-A in the Treatment of Chronic Daily Headache

Botulinum toxin type-A may be best suited for the treatment of CDH. Ondo et al conducted a double-blind study that showed patients that received BOTOX had significantly fewer days of headaches than those receiving a placebo.[34] Miller and Denny and Tepper et al concluded in a retrospective cohort analysis that most patients with refractory headache received a good response.[35,36] More recently, Mathew et al conducted a randomized, placebo-controlled study of 279 placebo nonresponders who enjoyed more headache-free

Figure 7-1. BOTOX injection sites for migraine headache. Total dose 60 to 200 units (see text). (Illustration by Lauren Shavell of Medical Imagery.)

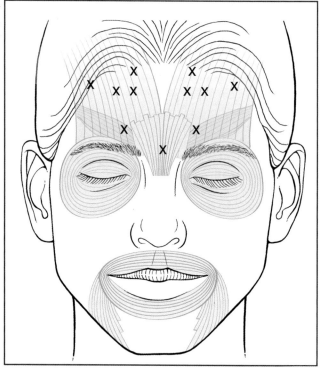

days when treated with BOTOX than a placebo.[37] More patients had a decrease from baseline of 50% or greater in frequency of headache days when treated with BOTOX.[37]

Although many of the previous studies show promising results for the use of botulinum toxin type-A for the treatment of different headache disorders, there is undoubtedly controversy even among experts in the field. Part of the reason for this controversy and conflicting results may be attributable to the placebo effect of a partially invasive treatment or a universally established dose or injection site protocol.

Procedures for Administration of Botulinum Toxin Type-A for Migraines

The method of administering and total dose given of botulinum toxin type-A will likely affect clinical outcome. It is also important to start with the correct diagnosis. Candidates for botulinum toxin type-A outlined by Blumenfeld et al include patients with disabling primary headaches; patients who have failed to respond to or have unacceptable side effects from conventional treatments; patients in whom standard preventative treatments are contraindicated; patients misusing or overusing medications; or patients with coexistent jaw, head, or neck muscle spasm.[38]

At this time, most experienced injectors use between 60 and 200 units. A typical injection pattern for migraine headache without significant cervical or occipital involvement is seen in Figure 7-1. Figure 7-2 represents commonly used treatment areas in the neck and back. The most important region seems to be the corrugator-procerus complex (glabellar region), and typically this area would receive about 15 units, with another 15 to 20 units

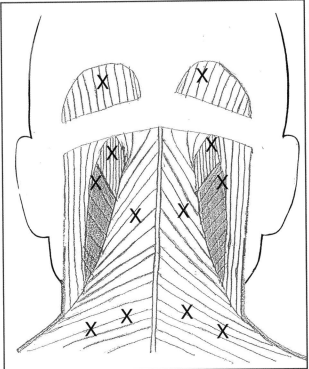

Figure 7-2. BOTOX injection sites for migraine headache. Total dose 60 to 200 units (see text).

across the frontalis, and at least 15 units in each temporalis at 3 or more sites. Use in the occipital and cervical region requires more experience and a careful history and examination for focal tenderness, trigger points, and recognition of abnormal head posture to determine the amount and location for injections.

To properly administer BOTOX for the treatment of headache, the needle is inserted below the dermis to ensure proper placement into the underlying muscle. The angle of insertion of the needle will vary by location. When injecting into the glabellar region, the needle should be inserted at an angle that is 45 degrees to 60 degrees from the skin surface directed superiorly away from the orbital rim (Figure 7-3). This should reduce the risk of upper eyelid ptosis that can result from BOTOX diffusing behind the orbital septum and weakening the levator palpebrae superioris muscle. When injecting the other muscle groups, including the frontalis, temporalis, occipitalis, and splenius capitus, the angle of needle insertion is typically 90 degrees or perpendicular to the skin surface (Figure 7-4).

While dilution of BOTOX with the saline vehicle may range from 100 units/mL (1 cc of diluent) to 12.5 units/mL (8 ccs of diluent), most headache injectors use 2 mL or 4 mL of diluent, resulting in 5 units/0.1 mL or 2.5 units/0.1 mL. We prefer the more dilute form for headache therapy because it theoretically allows for greater diffusion of toxin (see Table 4-1). A 30-gauge needle should be used for all injections unless there is a need for deep neck penetration. EMG guidance does not appear to have any role in the treatment of headache with botulinum toxin type-A.

Side effects of botulinum toxin type-A in the treatment of headache are not common. Ptosis is sometimes seen with inexperienced injectors who fail to avoid the central portion of the supraorbital region. Localized weakness may occur with injections into the neck, and patients may occasionally benefit from the use of a cervical collar for several weeks. Pain at the injection site is usually short lived, but it may last for weeks. Bruising and

Figure 7-3. Injections in the glabellar region should be performed with the needle inserted at an angle that is 45 degrees to 60 degrees from the skin surface and below the dermis to ensure proper placement into the underlying muscle. (Illustration by Lauren Shavell of Medical Imagery.)

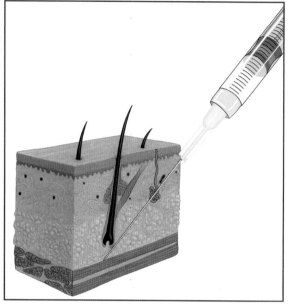

Figure 7-4. Injections in the forehead should be performed with the needle inserted at an angle that is 90 degrees from the skin surface and below the dermis to ensure proper placement into the underlying frontalis muscle. (Illustration by Lauren Shavell of Medical Imagery.)

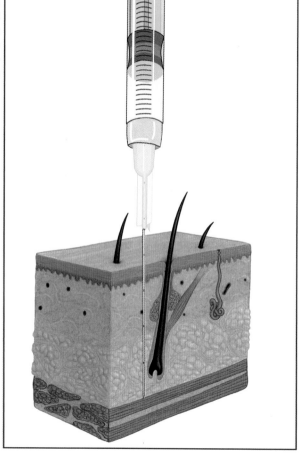

pain can be minimized with the use of 30-gauge needles and ice pack application before injection (see Figure 4-9).

Botulinum toxin type-B (MYOBLOC) has not been studied in the use of headache. While the target protein at the neuromuscular junction is different from type-A, botulinum toxin type-B works in much the same way as type-A and is likely to show efficacy similar to type-A. Anecdotally, MYOBLOC is said to cause more burning at the injection site because of its acidic diluent, and it also causes dry mouth at higher doses.

Summary

There is increasing evidence that botulinum toxin is beneficial in the treatment of migraine and possibly in TTHs. The current evidence is still not definitive, but 4 large, blinded, placebo-controlled studies are forthcoming, and these may lead to FDA approval for the treatment of migraine in the next several years. Increasing research suggests complex mechanisms of action that may be applicable to treatment of pain in other areas. While side effects of these injections are minimal, cost/benefit concerns and reimbursement issues remain the most significant barriers to usage.

References

1. Lipton RB, Stewart WF, Diamond S, et al. Prevalence and burden of migraine in the United States: data from the American migraine study II. *Headache*. 2002;41(7);646-657.
2. Hu XH, Markson LE, Lipton RB, et al. Burden of migraine in the United States: disability and economic costs. *Arch Intern Med*. 1999;159:813-818.
3. McCaig LF, Burt CW. National hospital ambulatory medical care survey: 1999 emergency department summary. Advance Data From Vital and Health Statistics: no. 320 Hyattsville, Md: National Center for Health Statistics; 2001. Available at: http://www.cdc.gov/nchs/data/ad/ad320.pdf. Accessed May 3, 2007.
4. Barron R, Carlsen J, Duff SB, Burk C. Estimating the cost of an emergency room visit for migraine headache. *J Med Econ*. 2003;6:1-11.
5. Binder WJ, Brin MF, Blitzer A, et al. Botulinum toxin type-A for treatment of migraine headaches: an open label study. *Otolaryngol Head Neck Surg*. 2000;123(6):669-676.
6. Boureau F, Joubert JM, Lasserre V, et al. Double-blind comparison of an acetaminophen 400 mg-codeine 25 mg combination versus aspirin 1000 mg and placebo in acute migraine attack. *Cephalalgia*. 1994;14:156.
7. Headache Classification Committee of the International Headache Society. Classification and diagnostic criteria for headache disorders, cranial neuralgia and facial pain. *Cephalalgia*. 2004;24(suppl 1):1-160.
8. Rasmussen BK, Olesen J. Epidemiology of headache. International association for the study of Pain. Technical Corner from the IASP Newsletter. March/April 1996. Available at: http://www.iasp-pain.org/TC96MarApr.htmL. Accessed May 3, 2007.
9. Smetana GW. The diagnostic value of historical features in primary headache syndromes: a comprehensive review. *Arch Intern Med*. 2000;160:2729-2737.
10. Sandrini G, Cecchini AP, Tassorelli C, Nappy G. Diagnostic issues in chronic daily headache. *Curr Pain Headache*. 2001;5:551-556.
11. Scher A, Stewart W, Liberman J, Lipton R. Prevalence of frequent headache in a population sample. *Headache*. 1997;38:497-506.
12. Pascual J, Colas R, Castillo J. Epidemiology of chronic daily headache. *Curr Pain Headache*. 2001;5:529-536.
13. Silberstein S, Lipton R. Chronic daily headache. *Curr Opin Neurol*. 2000;13:277-283.

14. Diener HC, Katasarva Z. Analgesic/abortive overuse and misuse in chronic daily headache. *Curr Pain Headache*. 2001;5:545-550.
15. Newman LC, Goadsby P, Lipton RB. Cluster and related headaches. *Med Clin North Am*. 2001;85:997-1016.
16. Kudrow L. Cluster headache: diagnosis and management. *Headache*. 1979;19:142.
17. Durham PL, Cady R, Cady R. Regulation of calcitonin gene-related peptide secretion from trigeminal nerve cells by botulinum toxin type-A: implications for migraine therapy. *Headache*. 2004;44:35-43.
18. Lauritzen M. Cerebral blood flow in migraine and cortical spreading depression. *Acta Neurol Scand Suppl*. 1987;76:1-40.
19. Rollnik JD, Karst M, Fink M, Dengler R. Botulinum toxin type-A and EMG: a key to the understanding of chronic TTH. *Headache*. 2001;41:985.
20. Spierings EL. Headache continuum: concept and supporting evidence from recent study of chronic daily headache. *Clin J Pain*. 2001;17:337.
21. Bartleson JD. Transient and persistent neurological manifestations of migraine. *Stroke*. 1984;15:383.
22. May A, Bahra A, Buchel C, Frackowiak RS, Goadsby PJ. Hypothalamic activation in cluster headache attacks. *Lancet*. 1998;352:723-725.
23. Martigononi E, Solomon S. The complex chronic headache, mixed headache and drug overuse. In: Olesen J, Tfelt-Hansen P, Welch KM, eds. *The Headache*. New York: Raven; 1993:849.
24. Winner P, Ricalde O, Le Force B, et al. A double blind study of sub-cutaneous dihydroergotamine vs subcutaneous sumatriptan in the treatment of acute migraine. *Arch Neurol*. 1996;53:180.
25. Tfelt-Hansen P, De Vries P, Saxena PR. Triptans in migraine: a comparative review of pharmacology, pharmacokinetics and efficacy. *Drugs*. 2000;60:1259.
26. Raskin NH. Repetitive intravenous dihydroergotamine as therapy for intractable migraine. *Neurology*. 1986;36:995.
27. Kudrow L. Response of cluster headache attacks to oxygen inhalation. *Headache*. 1981;1:4.
28. Treatment of acute cluster headache with sumatriptan. The Sumatriptan Cluster Headache Study Group. *N Engl J Med*. 1991;325:322.
29. Barrientos N, Chana P. Efficacy and safety of botulinum toxin A (BOTOX) in the prophylactic treatment of migraine (abstract). *Headache*. 2002;42:452.
30. Eross EG, Dodick DW. The effects of botulinum toxin type-A on disability in episodic and chronic migraine. *Headache*. 2002;42(5):S108.2.
31. Smuts JA, Baker MK, Smuts HM, et al. Prophylactic treatment of chronic TTH using botulinum toxin type-A. *Eur J Neurol*. 1999;52(suppl 2):A202.
32. Schulte-Mattler WJ, Krack P. Treatment of chronic TTH with botulinum toxin A: a randomized, double-blind, placebo-controlled multicenter study. *Pain*. 2004;109:110-114.
33. Padberg M, de Bruijn SFTM, de Haan RJ, Tavy DLJ. Treatment of chronic TTH with botulinum toxin: a double-blind, placebo-controlled trial. *Cephalalgia*. 2004;24:675-680.
34. Ondo WG, Vuong KD, Derman HS. Botulinum toxin A for chronic daily headache: a randomized placebo-controlled, parallel design study. *Cephalalgia*. 2004;24:60-65.
35. Miller T, Denny L. Retrospective cohort analysis of 48 chronic headache patients treated with botulinum toxin type-A (BOTOX) in a combination fixed injection site and follow the pain protocol. *Headache*. 2002;42:389-463.
36. Tepper SJ, Bigal ME, Sheftell FD, Rapoport A. Botulinum neurotoxin type-A in the preventive treatment of refractory headache: a review of 100 consecutive cases. *Headache*. 2004;44:794-800.
37. Mathew NT, Frishberg BM, Gawel M, et al. Botulinum toxin type-A (BOTOX) for the prophylactic treatment of chronic daily headache: a randomized double-blind, placebo controlled trial. *Headache*. 2005;45:293-307.
38. Blumenfeld A, Binder W, Silberstein SD, Blitzer A. Procedures for administering botulinum toxin type-A for migraine and TTH. *Headache*. 2003;43:884-891.

Bibliography

Anderson PG, Jespersen LT. Dihydroergotamine nasal spray in the treatment of attacks of cluster headache: a double-blind trial vs. placebo. *Cephalalgia*. 1986;6:51.

Brin M, Swope D, O'Brien C, Abbasi C, Pogoda J. BOTOX for migraine: double-blind, placebo-controlled, region-specific evaluation. *Cephalalgia*. 2000;20:421-422.

Coleman I, Brown MD, Innes GD, et al. Parenteral metoclopramide for acute migraine: meta-analysis of randomized controlled trials. *BMJ*. 2004;329:1369.

Conway S, Delplanche C, Crowder J, Rothrock J. BOTOX therapy for refractory chronic migraine. *Headache*. 2005;45:355-357.

Ekbom K. Lithium from cluster headache: review of literature and preliminary results of long term treatment. *Headache*. 1981;21:132.

Eross EF, Gladstone JP, Lewis S, Rogers R, Dodic DW. Duration of migraine is a predictor for response to botulinum toxin type-A. *Headache*. 2005;45:308-314.

Evers S, Vollmer-Haase J, Schwaag S, et al. Botulinum type-A in the prophylactic treatment of migraine: a randomized, double-blind placebo controlled, parallel design study. *Cephalalgia*. 2004;24:838-843.

Freund BJ, Schwartz M. Treatment of chronic cervical-associated headache with botulinum toxin type-A: a pilot study. *Headache*. 2000;40:231-236.

Graff-Radford SB. Migraine prophylaxis. *Clinics in Family Practice*. 2005;7(3):445-462.

Holroyd KA, O'Donnell FG, Stensland M, et al. Management of chronic TTH with tricyclic antidepressant mediation, stress management therapy and there combination: a randomized controlled trial. *JAMA*. 2001;285:2208.

Jarrar RG, Black DF, Dodick DW, Davis DH. Outcome of trigeminal nerve section in the treatment of chronic cluster headache. *Neurology*. 2003;60:1360.

Mathew NT. Transformed migraine, analgesic rebound, and other chronic daily headaches. *Neurol Clin*. 1997;15:167.

Rapoport A, Stang P, Gutterman DL, et al. Analgesic rebound headache in clinical practice: data from a physician survey. *Headache*. 1996;36:14.

Relja M. Treatment of TTH by local injection of botulinum toxin. *Eur J Neurol*. 1997;4 (Suppl 2):S71-S73.

Relja M. Treatment of TTH with botulinum toxin: 1-year follow-up. *Cephalalgia*. 2000;20:336.

Schim J. Effect of preventive treatment with botulinum toxin type-A on acute headache: medication usage in migraine patients. *Curr Med Res Opin*. 2004;20(1):49-53.

Silberstein S, Mathew N, Saper J, Jenkins S. Botulinum toxin type-A as a migraine preventive treatment. *Headache*. 2000;40:445-450.

Silberstein SD, Schulman EA, Hopkins MM. Repetitive intravenous DHE in the treatment of refractory headache. *Headache*. 1990;30:334.

CHAPTER 8

Cosmetic Applications of Botulinum Toxin

William J. Lipham, MD, FACS

BOTOX has been FDA approved in the United States since December 1989 for the treatment of a variety of functional disorders, including strabismus, hemifacial spasm, and blepharospasm; however, it was not until recently that it received FDA approval for the cosmetic reduction of glabellar frown lines.[1] In the early 1990s, ophthalmologist Jean Carruthers noted that patients who had received multiple treatments of BOTOX for blepharospasm benefited from a reduction in the appearance of their "frown" lines or glabellar furrows when BOTOX had been used to inactivate the central brow depressors. This initial observation led both her and her husband, Alastair Carruthers, a dermatologist, to perform BOTOX injections into the glabellar region of their patients for purely cosmetic indications. They reported their results in 1992 at the annual meeting of the American Academy of Dermatology and published the first paper on this subject the same year.[2] Their early findings led other investigators to begin treating additional muscle groups to similarly reduce the development of active lines of facial expression.[3,4] These additional regions included the lateral orbicularis oculi muscle to reduce crow's feet and the frontalis muscle to reduce transverse forehead lines as well as various muscles of the lower face and neck.[5-10]

Clinical success with BOTOX for wrinkle reduction has resulted in dramatically increased utilization of the substance for cosmetic purposes in the United States and abroad.[4,11-15] BOTOX—from its original use for wrinkle reduction in 1992 until April 15, 2002 when it was FDA approved for the treatment of glabellar furrows—had been used in an "off-label" fashion by physicians for cosmetic purposes. Throughout this time period, a broad range of specialists, including ophthalmologists, dermatologists, and facial plastic surgeons, integrated the use of botulinum toxin into their cosmetic armamentarium. Physicians in all of these disciplines frequently use botulinum toxin type-A alone as a minimally invasive procedure to reduce the appearance of active lines and wrinkles or in conjunction with other aesthetic procedures, including chemical peels, laser skin resurfacing, blepharoplasty surgery, and forehead and face-lifting procedures.[16]

Active or Mimetic Lines Versus Lines That Are Present "At Rest"

It is important to distinguish to both physicians and patients the difference between active or kinetic lines of facial expression and passive lines that are present at rest. Mimetic or kinetic lines develop through the repeated contraction of facial muscles that are responsible for creating a variety of facial expressions. Examples include vertical glabellar folds or "frown" lines, lateral orbicularis oculi rhytides or "smile" lines, and transverse forehead lines that develop from contraction of the frontalis muscle in an effort to elevate the brows. Botulinum toxin exerts its wrinkle-reducing effect by inactivating the muscles of facial expression that are responsible for the formation of these dynamic or mimetic lines.[17]

Repetitive facial expressions over a number of years eventually result in the formation of lines that are present "at rest" due to the breakdown and remodeling of collagen in the deeper dermis and subcutaneous tissue. For these individuals, inactivation of the muscles of facial expression with botulinum toxin will not yield as dramatic an effect because lines of facial expression are now present even when the muscles are at rest. For this reason, botulinum toxin injections for cosmetic wrinkle reduction are best suited for younger individuals who are starting to develop active lines of facial expression and would like to prevent the lines from becoming present at rest. The typical age range for this subset of patients is between 30 and 50 years of age.

For individuals who have lines that are present when their facial muscles are relaxed, alternative treatments may be considered. If the lines are fine and result primarily from a loss of skin elasticity, chemical peels or laser skin resurfacing may be the best options because these approaches promote epidermal turnover and tighten and smooth the underlying dermis.[18,19] In contrast, dermal filler agents, which include collagen as well as hyaluronic acid (HA) derivatives, are the best options to reduce the appearance of deeper lines that are present at rest. These compounds exert their effect by filling in and "plumping up" the underlying dermis to elevate the skin surface and reduce the depth of the wrinkle or line.[20,21] Laser skin resurfacing and chemical peels are excellent tools for facial rejuvenation; however, their application will not be discussed in this text, although the proper indications and administration of dermal filler agents will be covered in Chapter 9.

Clinical Evaluation

The easiest and most direct method to evaluate a patient with concerns about facial rhytides is to provide him or her with a hand mirror and ask him or her to identify the lines that he or she finds cosmetically unappealing (Figure 8-1). This will provide the physician with an opportunity to discuss the difference between active or mimetic lines and lines that are present "at rest," and allow him or her to develop a treatment strategy that best addresses the patient's concerns. As mentioned previously, it is important to understand and explain the differences between active or mimetic lines and lines that are present "at rest" so your patients have a better understanding of the indications and limitations for the variety of treatment options that exist.

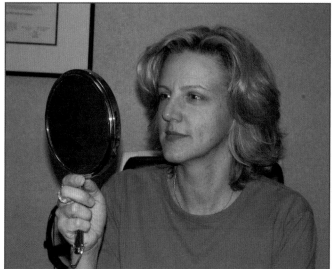

Figure 8-1. When evaluating a patient for cosmetic purposes, it is beneficial to provide him or her with a hand mirror to allow him or her to identify areas that he or she would like to discuss.

Suggested Dilution Protocols

BOTOX may be reconstituted with either 1 mL or 2 mL of sterile, nonpreserved saline to yield a concentration of 10 units/0.1 mL or 5 units/0.1 mL, respectively (see Chapter 4). For both functional and cosmetic purposes, I prefer to use a 3-mL syringe to reconstitute the lyophilized BOTOX with 2.2 mL of normal saline to provide a final concentration of approximately 5 units/0.1 mL. The additional 0.2 mL of saline is added to compensate for the volume of solution that is lost in the hub of the needle (usually 0.05 mL for each 1-mL syringe) from the 3 to 4 treatment areas that are typically obtained from a single vial of botulinum toxin. Reconstituting BOTOX in this manner provides volumes that are easy to work with because 2.5 to 5 units of BOTOX or 0.05 mL or 0.1 mL volumes are injected at each site in most instances, which is easy to perform with a 1-cc tuberculin syringe (Table 8-1).

While the manufacturers of Dysport recommend diluting each vial with 2.5 cc of sterile, nonpreserved saline, this provides a solution with a concentration of 20 units/0.1 cc, which yields a 4:1 ratio when compared to an equivalent volume of BOTOX. At present, there are conflicting reports that describe the ratio of Dysport units to BOTOX units, ranging from 3:1 to 4:1.[22-24] It has been the author's experience while working with Dysport in Asia that 3 Dysport units are clinically equivalent to 1 BOTOX unit for cosmetic purposes. These observations are consistent with a randomized, double-blinded study that was performed to determine the dose equivalency of Dysport and BOTOX for the treatment of cervical dystonia.[24] Since there are 500 units in each vial of Dysport, dose-volume equivalency at a 3:1 ratio with respect to BOTOX may be obtained by diluting each Dysport vial with 4.0 mL of sterile, nonpreserved saline (Table 8-2). For the remainder of this chapter, recommended doses of BOTOX and Dysport will be provided following these dilution protocols.

It should also be noted that the sterile, nonpreserved normal saline should be added slowly to the vial when reconstituting botulinum toxin. Care should be taken to hold onto the plunger of the syringe as it enters the vial since the lyophilized powder is maintained in a vacuum (see Chapter 4). If the normal saline is allowed to enter the vial rapidly, it will create

Table 8-1

Reconstitution Volumes of BOTOX and Dysport

BOTOX may be reconstituted with either 1 mL to 4 mL of sterile, nonpreserved saline to yield a variety of concentrations. I prefer to reconstitute the lyophilized BOTOX with 2.2 mL of normal saline to provide a final concentration of approximately 5 units per 0.1 cc (shown in bold/italic). The additional 0.2 mL of saline is added to compensate for the volume of solution that is lost in the hub (usually 0.05 mL per 1-cc syringe) from the 3 to 4 treatment areas that are typically obtained from a single vial of botulinum toxin.

Reconstitution Volume	BOTOX Units/0.1 mL	BOTOX Units/0.05 mL
1.0 mL	10	5
2.0 mL	5	2.5
2.2 mL	*4.5*	*2.25*
2.5 mL	4	2
4.0 mL	2.5	1.25

Table 8-2

Reconstitution of BOTOX and Dysport for Cosmetic Purposes

Different studies have shown that Dysport dose equivalents to BOTOX range from a 3:1 to 4:1 ratio. For this reason, lower concentrations should be employed for cosmetic purposes to avoid potential complications from injecting large doses of Dysport.

	BOTOX	Dysport
Vial contents	100 units	500 units
Reconstitution volume	2.5 mL	4 mL
Injection concentration	4 units/0.1 cc	12 units/0.1 cc
Ratio Dysport:BOTOX	–	3:1

significant turbulence, causing the light chains and heavy chains to disassociate, and will render the botulinum toxin inactive.

Treatment of Glabellar Furrows

As noted previously, the first area to be successfully treated and FDA approved with botulinum toxin for cosmetic purposes was the glabellar region. The central brow depressors consist of the procerus muscle, depressor supercilii, and corrugator muscle complex (see Figure 3-4).[25] Contraction of the procerus muscle over time produces a transverse line

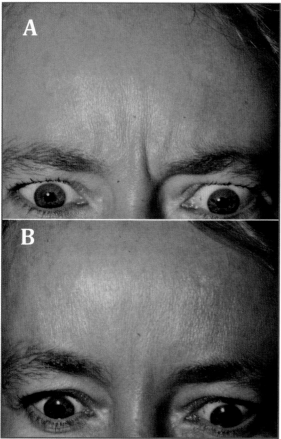

Figure 8-2. Inactivation of the central brow depressors induces a smoothing or softening effect between the eyebrows and above the nasal bridge as seen in this patient (A) prior to botulinum toxin type-A administration and (B) 2 weeks following injection.

that is located immediately below the glabellar region above the nasal bridge (see Figure 3-5).[26] In contrast, the corrugator muscle, along with the depressor supercilii muscle, is responsible for the development of vertical glabellar furrows or "frown" lines that are located medial to the brow cilia (see Figure 3-6).

The corrugator muscle lies deep to the procerus as well as the frontalis muscle. It originates from the superomedial aspect of the orbital rim just nasal to the brow cilia. It then passes laterally through the galeal fat pad above the brow to insert into the superficial dermis within the central aspect of the eyebrow. The depressor supercilii muscle is located just below the corrugator muscle and similarly contributes to the creation of glabellar furrows or "frown" lines.[25] When botulinum toxin is administered into the region of the corrugator muscle, it simultaneously weakens the depressor supercilii muscle because they lie in close juxtaposition and can be conceptualized as a single functional entity. Inactivation of all 5 central brow depressor muscles induces a smoothing or softening effect between the eyebrows and above the nasal bridge (Figure 8-2).

INJECTION TECHNIQUE

Prior to treatment, the patient is asked to produce a facial expression (typically a scowl) that will activate the central brow depressors to determine the proper dosage and distribution of botulinum toxin to be injected. This is best accomplished by providing the patient with a hand mirror and asking him or her to frown or "look angry" (see

Figure 8-3. Physician positioning for injection of glabellar furrows. It is easiest to stand to the patient's side so injections may be directed superiorly away from the orbital septum.

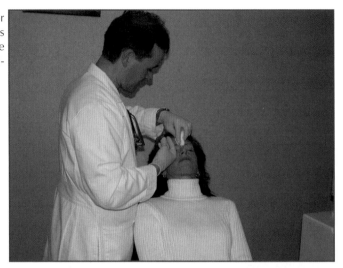

Figure 8-4. Injections in the glabellar region should be performed with the needle directed slightly caudad and away from the orbit to avoid inadvertent spread of the botulinum toxin behind the septum, which may weaken the extraocular muscles or levator palpebrae superioris and inadvertently induce diplopia and/or ptosis.

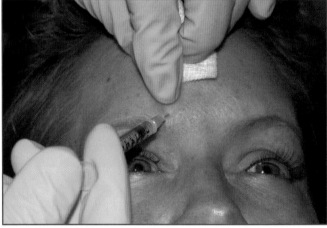

Figure 3-5). The intensity and strength of muscle contraction is then evaluated. It should be noted that there is significant variability between patients in both the volume of muscle and the strength of contraction. In addition, men typically have much greater muscle volume and strength compared to women, so dosing should be adjusted accordingly.

Injections can be conveniently performed in a clinic setting with the patient sitting in a reclining examination chair (Figure 8-3). It has been the author's experience that it is difficult to perform injections in a conventional chair because they lack head support and performing injections on a procedure bed is time consuming and cumbersome. A reclining clinic chair, however, provides excellent neck support for the patient when it is tilted backwards 25 degrees to 30 degrees from the upright position. To treat this area, it is best for the physician to stand at the patient's side so that the injections may be administered with the needle directed slightly superior to or away from the orbit to avoid inadvertent spread of the botulinum toxin behind the septum, which may weaken the extraocular muscles or levator palpebrae superioris and inadvertently induce diplopia and/or ptosis (Figure 8-4). To properly administer BOTOX into the glabellar region, the needle should be inserted at angle that is 45 degrees to 60 degrees from the skin surface and directed superiorly away from the orbital rim. The needle is inserted below the dermis to ensure

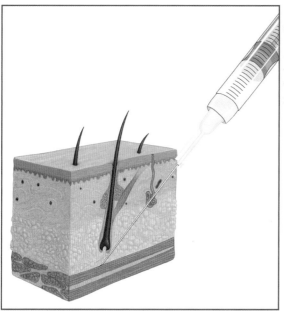

Figure 8-5. Injections in the glabellar region should be performed with the needle inserted at an angle that is 45 degrees to 60 degrees from the skin surface and below the dermis to ensure proper placement into the underlying muscle. (Illustration by Lauren Shavell of Medical Imagery.)

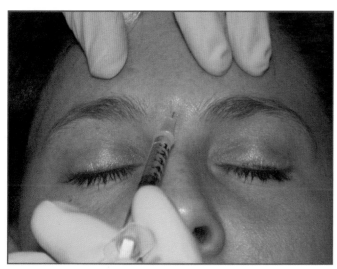

Figure 8-6. The procerus muscle may be inactivated with either 2.5 to 5 units of BOTOX or 7.5 to 15 Dysport units as a single injection in the central body of the muscle.

proper placement into the underlying muscle (Figure 8-5). This should reduce the risk of upper eyelid ptosis that can result from BOTOX diffusing behind the orbital septum and weakening the levator palpebrae superioris muscle. Additional suggestions on how to correctly set up and perform botulinum toxin injections are covered under the section "Clinical Implementation" in Chapter 4 (see p. 30).

The procerus muscle is located between the glabellar furrows and runs vertically between the 2 "frown" lines. It originates from the inferior aspect of the galea aponeurotica to insert into the dorsum of the nasal bridge where it merges with the nasalis muscle. The procerus muscle may be inactivated with either 2.5 to 5 units of BOTOX or 7.5 to 15 Dysport units as a single injection in the central body of the muscle (Figure 8-6).

Five BOTOX units or 15 Dysport units may be given to the medial aspect of the corrugator muscle complex in most individuals (Figure 8-7). This injection site is located just

Figure 8-7. For most individuals, 5 BOTOX units or 15 Dysport units may be given to the medial aspect of the corrugator muscle complex, which is located just medial to the medial aspect of the brow or approximately 3 mm inside the medial canthus.

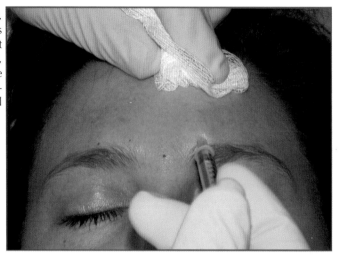

Figure 8-8. The lateral aspect of the corrugator muscle may be injected in a similar fashion depending on the strength and tone of the muscle. For most patients, 2.5 to 5 units of BOTOX or 7.5 to 15 units of Dysport may be administered to this area.

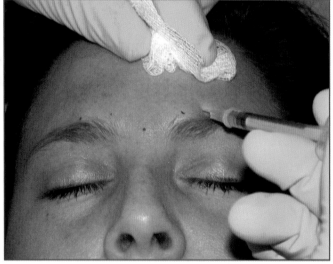

medial to the medial aspect of the brow or approximately 3 mm inside the medial canthus of the eye. Since the depressor supercilii and the corrugator muscle overlap in this region, a greater amount of BOTOX must be administered in this area to inactivate the depressor supercilii/corrugator complex.

The lateral aspect of the corrugator muscle may be injected in a similar fashion depending on the strength and tone of the muscle. For most patients, 2.5 to 5 units of BOTOX or 7.5 to 15 units of Dysport may be administered to the lateral aspect of the corrugator muscle complex (Figure 8-8). The exact location of the injection is dependent on the area of muscle contraction, but it usually corresponds to an area superior to the brow cilia and directly above the medial aspect of the pupil. It is important to carefully observe the muscle contraction in this region to inactivate the lateral aspect of this muscle. Total injection doses for the central brow depressors, therefore, range from 17.5 to 25 units of BOTOX or 52.5 to 75 units of Dysport, depending on the individual's muscle volume and strength of contraction (Figure 8-9).

The epidermis and dermis are quite thick in the glabellar region and are approximately 280 μm to 300 μm in depth. In addition, the procerus and corrugator muscles lie beneath

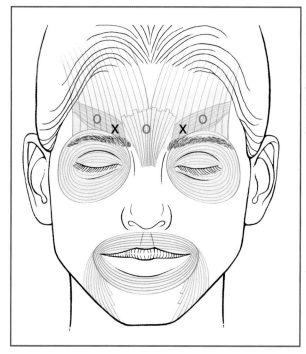

Figure 8-9. Reduction of glabellar furrows: Each "X" marked in black typically requires 5 BOTOX units or 15 Dysport units. Each "O" marked in gray indicates areas that may be given a variable amount of BOTOX depending on muscle strength using 2.5 to 5 units BOTOX units or 7.5 to 15 Dysport units accordingly. (Illustration by Lauren Shavell of Medical Imagery.)

subcutaneous brow fat while the depressor supercilii lies beneath the corrugator muscle itself. For these reasons, the 30-gauge needle should be inserted at least 3 mm to 6 mm below the skin surface, depending on the muscle volume and thickness of the tissue. Prior to injection, the muscle should be palpated to determine its thickness and volume in order to determine the depth of the injection to ensure its proper intramuscular location. Care should be taken to avoid inserting the needle into the underlying periosteum because this causes significant discomfort and incorrectly administers the botulinum toxin into a muscular region, resulting in diminished clinical effect.

Complications: Glabellar Frown Lines

The most common complication of injections in the glabellar area is upper lid ptosis due to diffusion of the toxin through the orbital septum and weakening of the levator muscle. Injection of lower volumes (ie, higher concentrations) decreases the amount of toxin diffusion and reduces the risk of ptosis. This occurs between 2 and 10 days after the injection and persists for up to 4 weeks. In order to avoid ptosis, injections should extend no further laterally than the mid pupillary line, and they should be at least 2 cm above the eyebrow.[27]

Transverse Forehead Lines

Horizontal forehead lines most often result as a compensatory mechanism to clear the superior visual field when it is compromised by brow ptosis, hooding dermatochalasis, upper lid ptosis, or a combination of the 3. In contrast to treating glabellar and "crow's feet" lines, which have very few functional consequences, treating forehead lines requires more consideration. When treating the frontalis muscle for cosmetic purposes, it is impor-

Figure 8-10. Inadvertent administration of botulinum toxin to the lateral brow in a woman may result in cosmetically unappealing flattening of the brow contour.

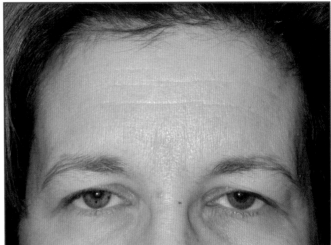

Figure 8-11. An aesthetically "ideal" female brow contour. The highest point of the brow should be located above the lateral canthus at the junction of the medial two-thirds and lateral one-third of the brow.

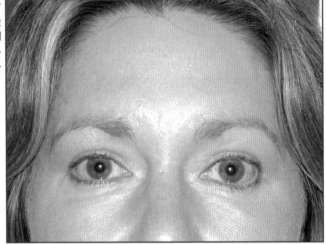

tant to avoid using large doses of botulinum toxin because this may result in generalized brow descent, giving the patient a tired or fatigued look (Figure 8-10).[28] For female patients, it is desirable to allow them to retain the ability to elevate the lateral aspect of their brow, as this will favor a cosmetically appealing brow contour. An aesthetically "ideal" female brow contour rises upwards with its highest point positioned above the lateral canthus at the lateral third of the brow (Figure 8-11).

While the treatment of glabellar furrows and periocular "crow's feet" consists of relatively uniform treatment patterns that can be easily modified, treatment of transverse forehead lines requires a more individualized approach. When evaluating a patient for reduction of transverse forehead lines, the patient should be asked to elevate his or her brows to determine the strength of the frontalis muscle as well as the location of the lines that are generated by forceful contraction (Figure 8-12). As described in Chapter 3, the frontalis muscle extends from the brow region superiorly and inserts into the galea aponeurotica at the hairline. There are very few muscle fibers in the central aspect of the forehead as this region consists primarily of facial connective tissue. For this reason, botulinum toxin exerts less of a clinical effect when injected into the central aspect of the forehead.

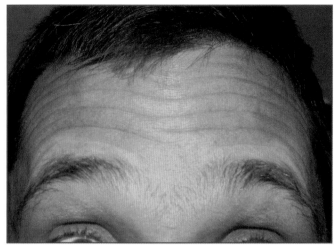

Figure 8-12. When evaluating a patient for reduction of transverse forehead lines, the physician should ask the patient to elevate his or her brows to determine the strength of the frontalis muscle as well as the location of the lines that are generated by forceful contraction.

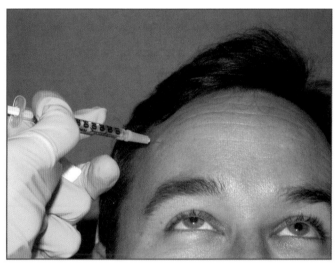

Figure 8-13. Using this approach, the needle is inserted into the skin surface perpendicularly because there is little risk of diffusion behind the orbital septum in this location.

Most authorities agree that injection of the transverse forehead region should be performed at least midway between the level of the brow cilia and hairline to reduce inadvertent diffusion into the central brow depressors.[29] While it may be reasonable to inject the lateral aspect of the frontalis muscle in men, it is generally advisable to avoid injecting this region in women to reduce the incidence of lateral brow ptosis, which is cosmetically undesirable.[28,30]

INJECTION TECHNIQUE

When performing forehead injections, I prefer to stand at the patient's side while he or she sits in a reclining examination chair tilted backwards at an angle of approximately 30 degrees to 45 degrees (see Figure 8-3). Using this approach, the needle is inserted through the skin surface perpendicularly, as there is little risk of diffusion behind the orbital septum in this location (Figure 8-13). In addition, the needle is inserted below the dermis to ensure proper placement into the underlying frontalis muscle (Figure 8-14). For most patients, 2 injections may be performed on either side of the forehead in the central area between the brow cilia and hairline. Typical injection doses consist of 2.5 to 5 units

Figure 8-14. Injections in the forehead should be performed with the needle inserted at an angle that is 90 degrees from the skin surface and below the dermis to ensure proper placement into the underlying frontalis muscle. (Illustration by Lauren Shavell of Medical Imagery.)

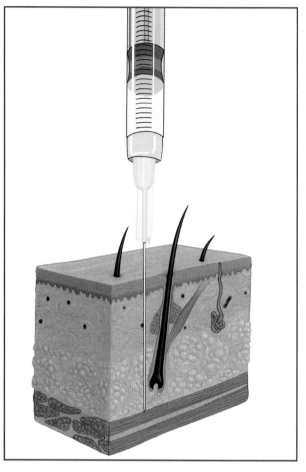

of BOTOX or 7.5 to 15 Dysport units to each area indicated with a black "X" (Figure 8-15). Centrally, the frontalis muscle contains fewer muscle fibers and may only require 2.5 to 5 BOTOX units or 7.5 to 15 Dysport units. In some individuals, it is better to inject only 2.5 units of BOTOX or 7.5 Dysport units at each injection site and spread the treatment injections over a greater area of the frontalis muscle to obtain a more uniform distribution (Figure 8-16).

Since the frontalis muscle is located beneath the thick skin of the scalp, the injections must be placed at least 4 mm to 5 mm below the skin surface to obtain a true intramuscular injection. Care should be taken to avoid injecting into or below the periosteum because this is painful for the patient and also reduces clinical effect. If you feel either the skull or periosteum while injecting, merely back the needle up approximately 3 mm to 4 mm before infiltrating the botulinum toxin.

Complications: Treatment of Forehead Lines

The primary complication that occurs when treating horizontal forehead lines is a state of inexpressivity or a mask-like appearance. In addition, brow ptosis, which is cosmetically unacceptable and sometimes visually significant, can occur. A quizzical or "cock-eyed" appearance can be seen when the medial forehead is paralyzed and lateral frontalis fibers remain functional. Performing injections at least 2 cm above the eyebrows

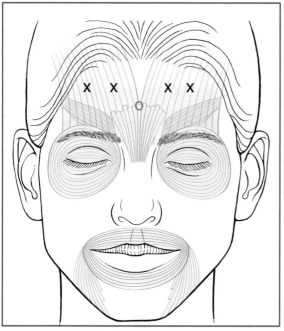

Figure 8-15. Treatment of transverse forehead lines: Injections should be performed at the "equator" of the brow midway between the brow cilia and hairline. Typical injection doses consist of 5 units of BOTOX or 15 Dysport units to each area indicated with a black "X." Centrally, the frontalis muscle contains fewer muscle fibers and may only require 2.5 to 5 BOTOX units or 7.5 to 15 Dysport units indicated with a gray "O." Injections should be avoided in the lateral forehead to prevent brow ptosis. (Illustration by Lauren Shavell of Medical Imagery.)

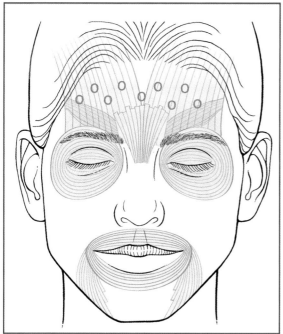

Figure 8-16. Alternate treatment pattern for treatment of transverse forehead lines: Typical injection doses consist of 2.5 units of BOTOX or 7.5 Dysport units to each area indicated with a gray "O." Injections should be avoided in the lateral forehead to prevent brow ptosis. (Illustration by Lauren Shavell of Medical Imagery.)

for the entire width of the frontalis muscle will help to avoid these complications. Assessing the full range of motion of the frontalis muscle prior to the injection will also allow complete treatment and prevent unwanted focal areas of residual function. If encountered, these complications are untreatable, but the patient can be reassured that they will resolve in 3 to 4 months.

Figure 8-17. Nonsurgical or botulinum toxin "browlift": Each "X" marked in black typically requires 5 BOTOX units or 15 Dysport units. Inactivation of the central brow depressors may be treated as described previously for inactivation of glabellar furrows. Lateral brow elevation is obtained by inactivating the superotemporal fibers of the orbicularis with a single injection of 5 BOTOX units or 15 Dysport units per side. (Illustration by Lauren Shavell of Medical Imagery.)

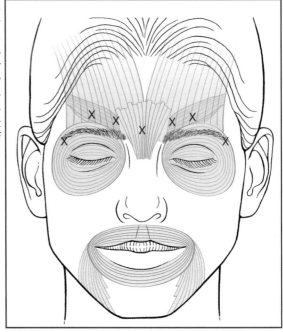

Nonsurgical or "BOTOX" Brow Lift

As described previously, the frontalis muscle serves as the sole elevator of the eyebrows while the corrugator, procerus, and orbicularis muscles are the brow depressors. Frankel et al demonstrated that the medial brow elevates when the corrugator muscle is injected with botulinum toxin type-A.[31] Huilgol et al then demonstrated mild elevation of the entire brow when both the corrugator and lateral orbital orbicularis are injected with botulinum toxin type-A (mean = 1 mm lift).[32] A typical injection pattern includes treatment of the central brow depressors as described above for treatment of glabellar furrows, with additional injections performed below the lateral brow cilia to inactivate the superotemporal aspect of the orbicularis muscle, which acts as the lateral brow depressor (Figure 8-17).

Huang et al provided a quantitative statistical analysis by injecting both the corrugator and orbicularis muscles, demonstrating elevation of the medial, central, and lateral eyebrows.[33] Injection of the brow depressors is unlikely to be effective in severe brow ptosis associated with involutional changes, but it offers an effective nonsurgical alternative for moderate brow ptosis.

Treatment of Orbicularis Rhytides or "Crow's Feet"

Contraction of the lateral orbicularis muscle is responsible for the creation of active lines or wrinkles that radiate from the lateral canthal angle, which are commonly referred to as "smile" lines or "crow's feet" (Figure 8-18). Although crow's feet lines are often associated with positive emotions such as smiling and laughing, they can contribute to a

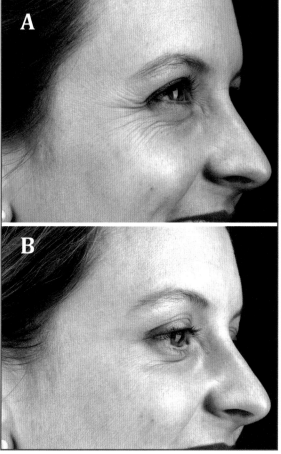

Figure 8-18. Contraction of the lateral orbicularis oculi muscle is responsible for the creation of active lines or wrinkles that radiate from the lateral canthal angle, which are commonly referred to as "smile" lines or "crow's feet." Injection of this area with botulinum toxin softens these lines as seen in this patient (A) prior to botulinum toxin administration and (B) 1 month after injection.

more aged appearance, especially when combined with photo-aged skin. As the skin in this region is quite thin (60 µm to 80 µm) most currently available dermal filler agents are incapable of reducing these lines effectively without inducing unwanted over correction. Since these are lines caused by active muscle contraction, they may be effectively treated with botulinum toxin injections. The injections may be distributed at either 2 or 3 locations along the lateral canthal angle.

INJECTION TECHNIQUE

To evaluate this area, the patient is asked to make an exaggerated smile in order to induce orbicularis muscle contraction. The examining physician should palpate the muscle during this maneuver to determine the volume and strength of muscular contraction.

Injections may be performed from a position directly above the patient's head with the needle directed away from the orbital septum (Figure 8-19). Alternatively, the physician may stand at the patient's side and instruct the patient to turn his or her head toward the physician to treat the contralateral side (Figure 8-20). Either injection technique will facilitate directing the stream of botulinum toxin type-A away from the orbital septum to reduce the risk of post-treatment ptosis or diplopia. In addition, the angle of injection is typically flatter than those performed in the glabellar region or forehead and is

Figure 8-19. Injections may be performed with the physician located directly above the patient's head to orient the needle away from the orbital septum to reduce the appearance of "crow's feet."

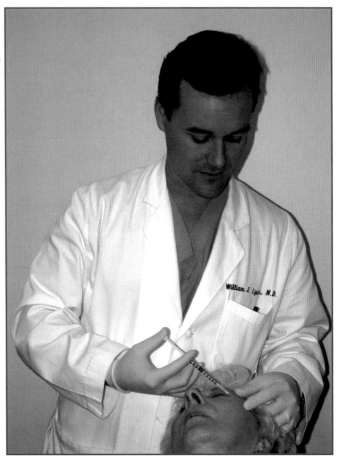

Figure 8-20. Alternatively, the physician may stand at the patient's side and instruct the patient to turn his or her head toward the physician to treat the contralateral side.

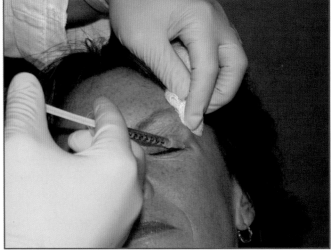

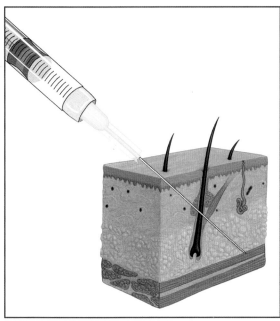

Figure 8-21. Injections to reduce the appearance of "crow's feet" or "smile" lines should be performed with the needle oriented at an angle that is 30 degrees from the skin surface. The tip of the needle is inserted immediately below the dermis to ensure diffusion and inactivation of the underlying orbicularis oculi muscle. (Illustration by Lauren Shavell of Medical Imagery.)

carried out at an angle of 30 degrees as compared to the more vertically oriented injections performed elsewhere. Since the skin is extremely thin in the lateral orbicularis region, injections are performed more superficially, approximately 1 mm to 2 mm below the skin surface, as there is very little or no subcutaneous fat beneath the dermis in this area (Figure 8-21).

If the person has light muscle volume and relatively weak contractile force, 2 injection sites may be used to inactivate this region. The injection sites are typically placed just outside the lateral edge of the orbital rim approximately 3 mm to 5 mm superior and inferior to the lateral canthal angle (Figure 8-22). The diameter of dispersion of botulinum toxin for each injection site is approximately 1 cm with the greatest treatment effect occurring within this area (Figure 8-23).

For individuals with greater orbicularis muscle volume or increased contraction strength, 3 injections per side may be performed. The first injection is placed in the same horizontal plane as the lateral canthal angle at or just lateral to the lateral orbital rim, which can be easily palpated (Figure 8-24). Two additional injections are placed superior and inferior to the initial injection (similar in location to the 2-injection-site-per-side technique) to soften the appearance of the lines in this area of muscle contraction (Figure 8-25).

When injecting individuals using 2 injection sites per side, I typically use 5 BOTOX units or 15 Dysport units per injection site (see Figure 8-23). For individuals with stronger muscle tone, the superior and inferior injections are typically performed with 5 BOTOX units per site or 15 Dysport units per site, while the central injection in the lateral canthal angle may consist of 2.5 to 5 BOTOX units or 7.5 to 15 Dysport units, depending on the amount of muscular contraction and muscle volume (see Figure 8-25).

Figure 8-22. For patients with less orbicularis oculi muscle volume and relatively weak contractile force, 2 injection sites may be used to inactivate this region. The injection sites are typically placed just outside the lateral edge of the orbital rim approximately 3 mm to 5 mm superior and inferior to the lateral canthal angle.

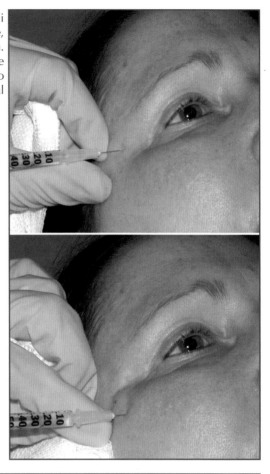

Figure 8-23. Two-injection-site technique for orbicularis rhytides or "crow's feet": Each "X" represents approximately 5 BOTOX units or 15 Dysport units per injection site. (Illustration by Lauren Shavell of Medical Imagery.)

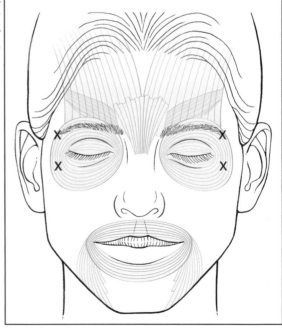

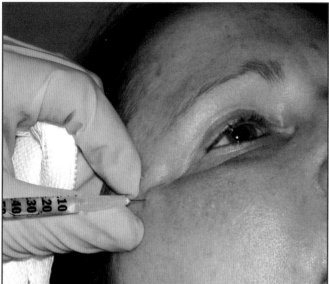

Figure 8-24. For individuals with greater orbicularis muscle volume or increased contraction strength, 3 injections per side may be performed. The first injection is placed in the same horizontal plane as the lateral canthal angle at or just lateral to the lateral orbital rim, which can be easily palpated.

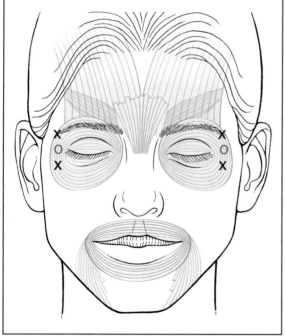

Figure 8-25. Three-injection-site technique for orbicularis rhytides or "crow's feet": Each black "X" represents approximately 5 BOTOX units or 15 Dysport units per injection site. The lateral canthal angle injections consist of either 2.5 to 5 BOTOX units or 7.5 to 15 Dysport units represented by a gray "O." (Illustration by Lauren Shavell of Medical Imagery.)

"Bunny" Lines

Some patients may present with transverse lines over their nasal bridge that they may find cosmetically unappealing. These lines are induced by contraction of the nasalis muscle and are commonly referred to as "bunny" lines (Figure 8-26). This muscle group is best treated with 2 to 3 low-dose botulinum toxin injections on either side of the nasal bridge corresponding to the location of the nasalis muscle whose anatomy is described in

Figure 8-26. Contraction of the nasalis muscle over time may cause transverse lines to develop over the patient's nasal bridge, which patients may find cosmetically unappealing. These lines are commonly referred to as "bunny" lines.

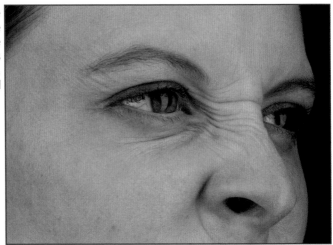

Figure 8-27. Injections to reduce the appearance of "bunny" lines should be performed with the needle inserted at an angle that is 45 degrees to 60 degrees from the skin surface and below the dermis to ensure proper placement into the underlying nasalis muscle. (Illustration by Lauren Shavell of Medical Imagery.)

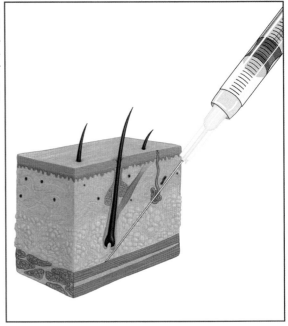

detail in Chapter 3. Injections should be performed with the needle inserted at an angle that is 45 degrees to 60 degrees from the skin surface and below the dermis to ensure proper administration into the underlying nasalis muscle (Figure 8-27). Typical injection doses range from 2.5 to 5 units of BOTOX and 7.5 to 15 units of Dysport (Figure 8-28). For initial treatments it is best to use the lower dose and titrate the dose upwards on subsequent sessions as indicated by effect. An additional injection may also be placed along the dorsum of the nasal bridge, but as there are fewer muscle fibers in this location, less clinical effect is obtained for an equivalent dose of botulinum toxin.

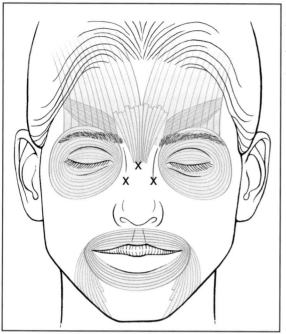

Figure 8-28. This nasalis muscle may be inactivated with 2 to 3 low-dose botulinum toxin injections on either side of the nasal bridge. Typical injection doses range from 2.5 to 5 units of BOTOX and 7.5 to 15 units of Dysport indicated with an "X." (Illustration by Lauren Shavell of Medical Imagery.)

Perioral Lines

Perioral or "smoker's" lines may be reduced with very low-dose placement of botulinum toxin into the perioral orbicularis oris muscle. Since such low doses are necessary to treat this area, it is recommended to dilute both BOTOX and Dysport with twice the normally recommended volumes of saline to obtain dilute solutions that provide lower doses of botulinum toxin for an equivalent volume of injection. Vertical upper lip wrinkles are caused by contraction of the orbicularis oris whose anatomy is described in Chapter 3 (see Figure 3-10). Typically, 1.25 to 2 units of BOTOX or 3.75 to 6 units of Dysport may be injected 5 mm above the vermilion border of the lip and placed approximately 1 cm to 2 cm apart to provide a total dose of no more than 5 to 8 units of BOTOX or 15 to 24 units of Dysport (Figure 8-29). Injections to reduce the appearance of "smoker's" lines should be performed with the needle inserted at an angle that is 90 degrees from the skin surface and below the dermis to ensure proper placement into the underlying orbicularis oris muscle (Figure 8-30). Initial dosing should be performed at the lower end of the suggested dose regimen and titrated upwards because the risk of paresis in this region is significant. Complications that may arise from administering too large a dose include difficulty whistling, smiling, or problems with pronunciation or mastication. Injections should always be performed using small volumes of botulinum toxin with high dilutions, and patients should be counseled that results might only be partial in effect and short in duration in order to avoid untoward complications.

Melomental or "Marionette" Lines

The downward turning lines at the lateral corners of the mouth may be reduced by chemodenervation of the depressor anguli oris, thereby allowing elevation of the corners

Figure 8-29. Perioral or "smoker's" lines may be reduced with very low-dose placement of botulinum toxin into the perioral orbicularis oris muscle. Typically 1.25 to 2 units of BOTOX or 3.75 to 6 units of Dysport may be injected 5 mm above the vermilion border of the lip and placed approximately 1 cm to 2 cm apart to provide a total dose of no more than 5 to 8 units of BOTOX or 15 to 24 units of Dysport. (Illustration by Lauren Shavell of Medical Imagery.)

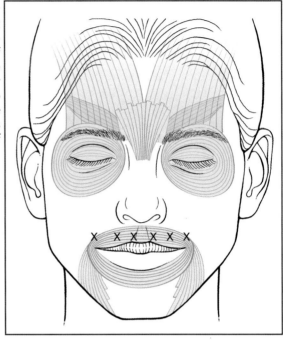

Figure 8-30. Injections to reduce the appearance of "smoker's" lines should be performed with the needle inserted at an angle that is 90 degrees from the skin surface and below the dermis to ensure proper placement into the underlying orbicularis oris muscle. (Illustration by Lauren Shavell of Medical Imagery.)

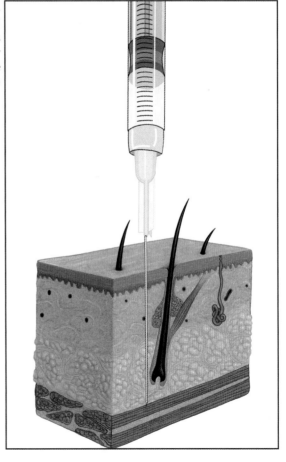

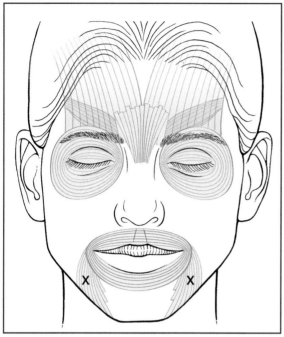

Figure 8-31. The downward turning lines at the lateral corners of the mouth may be reduced by chemodenervation of the depressor anguli oris muscle. Usually, 2.5 to 5 units of BOTOX or 7.5 to 15 units of Dysport are required to inactivate this muscle on each side. (Illustration by Lauren Shavell of Medical Imagery.)

of the mouth by the unopposed zygomaticus major and minor muscles. Platysmal injections may also be helpful to correct these lines because the platysma interdigitates with and contributes to the action of the depressor anguli oris muscle. The muscle may be identified by having the patient contract the muscle while looking into a hand mirror. The physician should palpate the contracting muscle to identify its location and mark the area with a surgical marker if necessary to confirm the proper site of injection. Usually 2.5 to 5 units of BOTOX or 7.5 to 15 units of Dysport are required to inactivate this muscle (Figure 8-31). Injections in this region should be performed with the needle inserted at an angle that is 90 degrees from the skin surface and below the dermis to ensure proper placement into the underlying depressor anguli oris muscle (Figure 8-32). While these injections may provide a good lift for the lateral corners of the mouth, they may produce transient problems with smiling or elocution, and injections into this region are not recommended for singers, musicians, or patients who use their perioral muscles with intensity (ie, scuba divers or trumpet players).

Platysmal Bands

While both hypertrophic platysmal bands and horizontal necklines have been improved with botulinum toxin injections, emphasis should be placed on the reduction of platysmal bands because the treatment of horizontal necklines is less predictable (Figure 8-33). Over time, the central platysmal bands thicken and contract, contributing to the formation of jowls and loss of neck definition. As described in Chapter 3, the platysma arises from the superficial fascia of the pectoralis and deltoid fascia and extends across the neck past the mandible. Some of the fibers insert into the mandible while others insert at the lateral oral commissure and contribute to a downward pulling action on the corners of the mouth. A variety of different injection techniques have been described in the medical literature.

Figure 8-32. Injections to reduce the appearance of melomental lines should be performed with the needle inserted at an angle that is 90 degrees from the skin surface and below the dermis to ensure proper placement into the underlying depressor anguli oris muscle. (Illustration by Lauren Shavell of Medical Imagery.)

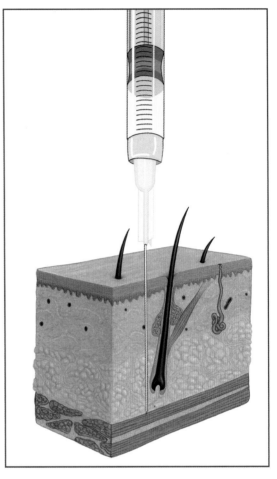

To determine the location of the injection, the patient is asked to contract the neck to reveal the platysmal band. The patient should push his or her forehead against the physician's hand to demonstrate the location of the bands nicely. Injections are then performed at 3 to 4 locations along each band for a total dose of 15 to 20 units of BOTOX or 45 to 60 units of Dysport with 5 BOTOX units or 15 Dysport units at each injection site (Figure 8-34). Usually no more than 4 bands are treated per session.

Complications associated with this region include transient edema, ecchymosis, and weakness of neck flexion. Rarely, recurrent laryngeal nerve weakness with associated hoarseness or dysphagia may develop 3 to 4 days after injection with doses in the range of 80 to 100 BOTOX units or 240 to 300 Dysport units.

Please see the following videos on the accompanying DVD:
Forehead and Frown Lines, Frown Lines, Chemical Browlift,
Smile and "Bunny" Lines, Forehead Lines, and Platysmal Bands.

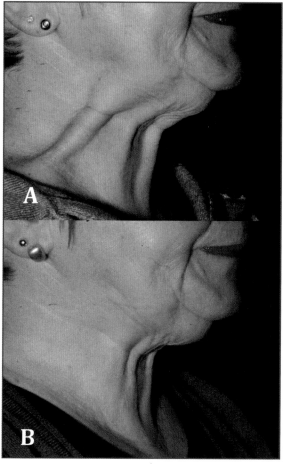

Figure 8-33. Over time, with repeated contraction, the central platysmal bands thicken and contribute to the formation of jowls and loss of neck definition. Injection of this area with botulinum toxin softens these lines as seen in this patient (A) prior to botulinum toxin type-A administration and (B) 1 month after injection.

References

1. Carruthers JA, Lowe NJ, Menter MA, et al. A multicenter, double-blind, randomized, placebo-controlled study of the efficacy and safety of botulinum toxin type A in the treatment of glabellar lines. *J Am Acad Dermatol.* 2002;46(6):840-849.
2. Carruthers JD, Carruthers JA. Treatment of glabellar frown lines with *C. botulinum*-A exotoxin. *J Dermatol Surg Oncol.* 1992;18(1):17-21.
3. Blitzer A, Brin MF, Keen MS, Aviv JE. Botulinum toxin for the treatment of hyperfunctional lines of the face. *Arch Otolaryngol Head Neck Surg.* 1993;119(9):1018-1022.
4. Keen M, Blitzer A, Aviv J, et al. Botulinum toxin type-A for hyperkinetic facial lines: results of a double-blind, placebo-controlled study. *Plast Reconstr Surg.* 1994;94(1):94-99.
5. Brandt FS, Bellman B. Cosmetic use of botulinum A exotoxin for the aging neck. *Dermatol Surg.* 1998;24(11):1232-1234.
6. Carruthers J, Carruthers A. BOTOX use in the mid and lower face and neck. *Semin Cutan Med Surg.* 2001;20(2):85-92.
7. Fagien S, Brandt FS. Primary and adjunctive use of botulinum toxin type A (BOTOX) in facial aesthetic surgery: beyond the glabella. *Clin Plast Surg.* 2001;28(1):127-148.
8. Kane MA. Nonsurgical treatment of platysmal bands with injection of botulinum toxin type-A. *Plast Reconstr Surg.* 1999;103(2):656-663; discussion 664-655.

Figure 8-34. Injections of the platysma muscle are performed at 3 to 4 locations along each band for a total dose of 15 to 20 units of BOTOX or 45 to 60 units of Dysport with 5 BOTOX units or 15 Dysport units at each injection site. Usually, no more than 4 bands are treated per session.

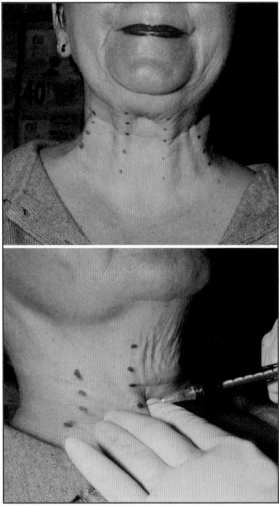

9. Sposito MM. New indications for botulinum toxin type A in treating facial wrinkles of the mouth and neck. *Aesthetic Plast Surg.* 2002;26(2):89-98.
10. Tanenbaum M. Aesthetic oculoplastic surgery. *Curr Opin Ophthalmol.* 1998;9(5):54-61.
11. Blitzer A, Binder WJ. Current practices in the use of botulinum toxin type-A in the management of facial lines and wrinkles. *Facial Plast Surg Clin North Am.* 2001;9(3):395-404.
12. Foster JA, Wulc AE, Holck DE. Cosmetic indications for botulinum A toxin. *Semin Ophthalmol.* 1998;13(3):142-148.
13. Klein AW. Treatment of wrinkles with BOTOX. *Curr Probl Dermatol.* 2002;30:188-217.
14. Markey AC. Botulinum A exotoxin in cosmetic dermatology. *Clin Exp Dermatol.* 2000;25(3):173-175.
15. Sarrabayrouse MA. Indications and limitations for the use of botulinum toxin for the treatment of facial wrinkles. *Aesthetic Plast Surg.* 2002;26(4):233-238.
16. Fagien S. BOTOX for the treatment of dynamic and hyperkinetic facial lines and furrows: adjunctive use in facial aesthetic surgery. *Plast Reconstr Surg.* 1999;103(2):701-713.
17. Foster JA, Barnhorst D, Papay F, Oh PM, Wulc AE. The use of botulinum A toxin to ameliorate facial kinetic frown lines. *Ophthalmology.* 1996;103(4):618-622.
18. Rohrer TE. Lasers and cosmetic dermatologic surgery for aging skin. *Clin Geriatr Med.* 2001;17(4): vii, 769-794.

19. Zimbler MS, Holds JB, Kokoska MS, et al. Effect of botulinum toxin pretreatment on laser resurfacing results: a prospective, randomized, blinded trial. *Arch Facial Plast Surg.* 2001;3(3):165-169.
20. Klein AW. Skin filling: collagen and other injectables of the skin. *Dermatol Clin.* 2001;19(3):ix, 491-508.
21. Naoum C, Dasiou-Plakida D. Dermal filler materials and botulin toxin. *Int J Dermatol.* 2001;40(10):609-621.
22. Lowe NJ. Botulinum toxin type A for facial rejuvenation: United States and United Kingdom perspectives. *Dermatol Surg.* 1998;24(11):1216-1218.
23. Nussgens Z, Roggenkamper P. Comparison of two botulinum-toxin preparations in the treatment of essential blepharospasm. *Graefes Arch Clin Exp Ophthalmol.* 1997;235(4):197-199.
24. Odergren T, Hjaltason S, Kaakkola S, Solders G, Hanko J, et al. A double blind, randomized, parallel group study to investigate the dose equivalence of Dysport and BOTOX in the treatment of cervical dystonia. *J Neurol Neurosurg Psychiatry.* 1998;64(1):6-12.
25. Cook BE, Jr, Lucarelli MJ, Lemke BN. Depressor supercilii muscle: anatomy, histology, and cosmetic implications. *Ophthal Plast Reconstr Surg.* 2001;17(6):404-411.
26. Pribitkin EA, Greco TM, Goode RL, Keane WM. Patient selection in the treatment of glabellar wrinkles with botulinum toxin type A injection. *Arch Otolaryngol Head Neck Surg.* 1997;123(3):321-326.
27. Matarasso SL. Complications of botulinum A exotoxin for hyperfunctional lines. *Dermatol Surg.* 1998;24(11):1249-1254.
28. Carucci JA, Zweibel SM. Botulinum A exotoxin for rejuvenation of the upper third of the face. *Facial Plast Surg.* 2001;17(1):11-20.
29. Koch RJ, Troell RJ, Goode RL. Contemporary management of the aging brow and forehead. *Laryngoscope.* 1997;107(6):710-715.
30. Wieder JM, Moy RL. Understanding botulinum toxin: surgical anatomy of the frown, forehead, and periocular region. *Dermatol Surg.* 1998;24(11):1172-1174.
31. Frankel AS, Kamer FM. Chemical browlift. *Arch Otolaryngol Head Neck Surg.* 1998;124(3):321-323.
32. Huilgol SC, Carruthers A, Carruthers JD. Raising eyebrows with botulinum toxin. *Dermatol Surg.* 1999;25:373-375.
33. Huang W, Rogachefsky AS, Foster JA. Browlift with botulinum toxin. *Dermatol Surg.* 2000;26(1):55-60.

CHAPTER 9

Cosmetic Filler Agents

Gregg S. Gayre, MD; David R. Jordan, MD;
and William J. Lipham, MD, FACS

The notion of facial rejuvenation through the injection of filler agents is certainly not new. Over the years, many substances, including mineral oil, paraffin, and liquid silicone, have been utilized as soft tissue fillers in an effort to improve soft tissue imperfections. Most of these substances were ultimately abandoned due to a high incidence of complications, including chronic edema, lymphadenopathy, granuloma formation, scarring, and ulcer formation. Currently, there has been a renewed interest in injectable fillers as more and more patients seek nonsurgical means for correcting age-related changes to their facial skin. One significant factor in this increased interest in injectable fillers has been the popularity that BOTOX has achieved.[1] BOTOX, which inhibits wrinkles caused by the muscles of facial expression, functions ideally in the upper face; however, its success in the lower face has thus far been limited. Filler substances serve as an attractive adjunctive therapy to BOTOX for the management of facial wrinkles, particularly in the lower face where the utilization of BOTOX is limited.

There are 2 basic types of wrinkles or rhytides: dynamic and static.[2] They may occur separately or in combination. Dynamic wrinkles appear within the skin due to repeated contracture by the underlying muscles of facial expression. Static rhytides appear regardless of facial dynamics and are due both to intrinsic changes in the components of the dermal ground substance and to exogenous changes brought about by such factors as smoking, gravity, and sun exposure.[3] The formation of both dynamic and static wrinkles is influenced by the quality of the natural collagen support layer within the dermal layers of the skin.

For the most part, dynamic rhytides and many combination rhytides are best treated by BOTOX injections, particularly in the upper face. However, for deeper wrinkles and furrows that do not resolve with BOTOX treatment alone, a filler substance used in combination with BOTOX may enhance the overall treatment outcome. In the lower face, injectable fillers often serve as the treatment of choice when treating both dynamic and static wrinkles. Although caution is indicated when using BOTOX in the lower face, it may serve a useful role in enhancing the treatment outcome of injectable fillers through its ability to reduce the stress imparted on the treated skin by the underlying muscles of facial expression.

The selection of the proper filler substance can be difficult. New products are continuously introduced, often with great excitement, but they all too frequently fail to fulfill the promise of a better injectable filler. The ideal tissue filler must be biocompatible, noncarcinogenic, and nonteratogenic. It should be nonmigratory and free of adverse reactions. It must be inexpensive, easy to use, widely available; should require little preparation; and provide predictable results. It should be natural looking, nonpalpable, long lasting, and require minimal recovery time.[4-11] Although no currently available injectable substance possesses all of these attributes, many new options exist that provide satisfactory results and excellent safety profiles.

Since the publication of the first edition of this text in 2004, a broad range of new filler agents has become available for use in the United States. In addition to bovine and human collagen, a wide variety of HA fillers has become FDA approved for aesthetic use. In addition to volume augmentation agents like collagen and HA fillers, a new class of fibroblast stimulator products—including poly-l-lactic acid (PLLA) (Sculptra™ [sanofi-aventis, Paris, France])—and calcium hydroxyapatite microspheres (Radiesse® [BioFirm Medical, Inc, San Mateo, Calif])—have also entered the market. Finally, a new permanent filler agent composed of polymethylmethacrylate (PMMA) microspheres, ArteFill® (Artes Medical, San Diego, Calif), has been recently FDA approved for the treatment of nasolabial folds.

To better conceptualize and organize the wide array of filler agents that is currently used in clinical practice, it is useful to categorize dermal fillers according to their physical properties and duration of effect. There are essentially 3 subsets of dermal filler agents available on the market. These include temporary biodegradable agents that last less than 1 year, semipermanent biodegradable agents that last 1 to 2 years, and permanent nonbiodegradable agents that last more than 2 years. The compounds that are in current clinical practice at the time of publication and their associated trade names are summarized in Table 9-1.

Temporary Biodegradable Compounds

This group of injectable fillers works by increasing volume in the area of administration and typically lasts less than 1 year. In the past few years, there has been a dramatic shift from the use of collagen-based compounds to HA fillers.[7,12-15] HA fillers have 2 main advantages over their collagen-based counterparts. The incidence of allergic reaction to HA products is significantly less than that of bovine collagen, and the duration of effect is superior with HA products when compared to both bovine and human collagen. The demand for bovine collagen has declined significantly since skin testing is required prior to clinical use. Human collagen, however, still has a role in certain applications and is an excellent agent for treatment of horizontal forehead lines and defining the vermilion border of the lips. In contrast, HA compounds work better for lip and nasolabial volume augmentation. As such, both agents are complementary and work well in conjunction with one another.

Bovine and Human Collagen

Collagen is the most abundant protein in the body, and much of the normal human dermis is composed of the collagen proteins. Collagen proteins are trimers involving 3 individual polypeptide chains, known as alpha chains. Each alpha chain is composed of about 1000 amino acids, with glycine occupying every third position. About 96% of the collagen molecule is helical, and these helices are attached to nonhelical telopeptides at

Table 9-1

Current Compounds Used in Clinical Practice

Temporary Biodegradable (<1 Year)	Semipermanent Biodegradable (1 to 2 Years)	Permanent Nonbiodegradable (>2 Years)
Collagen compounds Bovine collagen (Zyderm 1 and Zyderm 2/Zyplast) Human collagen (Cosmo-Derm/CosmoPlast)	Calcium hydroxyapatite (Radiesse) PLLA (Sculptra)	Silicone (SILIKON 1000) PMMA spheres (ArteFill)
HA compounds Restylane and Perlane Hylaform/Hylaform Plus Captique Puragen/Puragen Plus Juvéderm Ultra and Juvéderm Ultra Plus (United States) Juvéderm 18/24/30/24hv/ 30hv (Europe and Asia)	Cadaveric fascia lata (Fascian)	

the amino and carboxyl ends. In the human body, collagen molecules are cross-linked to form collagen fibrils, which then associate to form collagen fibers. Several types of collagen exist in humans. The types of collagen differ in regard to their combinations of alpha chains. Normal human dermal collagen is roughly 80% type I collagen and 20% type III collagen.[16,17]

It is the responsibility of the treating physician to counsel prospective patients about the risks and benefits of injectable collagen therapy prior to treatment. In addition, it is important to notify the patient of the cost of the implant material and the need for touch-up treatments.[18,19] It should be explained that corrections of 70% to 85% of the depression may constitute a good result, depending on the deformity. The patient must understand that effect of treatment is often a significant improvement in the deformity but not a complete resolution. Proper patient education, as well as realistic patient expectations of both the expected results and cost involved, are more likely to result in higher patient satisfaction, and a satisfied patient is 3 times more likely to continue treatment.

Bovine Collagen

When the first edition of this text was published in 2004, the single most popular form of injectable collagen was derived from bovine collagen.[19-21] The demand for this agent, however, has declined rapidly due to the emergence of new nonanimal stabilized HA compounds (NASHA). Unlike bovine collagen, which requires skin testing prior to aesthetic use, both human collagen and HA compounds can be used without prior skin testing since the incidence of allergic reaction is very low.[7,16] In the United States, injectable bovine collagen is manufactured under the trade name Zyderm® and Zyplast®, which were recently purchased by Allergan Incorporated.

Figure 9-1. Zyderm 1® collagen implants are purified fibrillar suspensions of bovine collagen, 3.5% by weight. (Reprinted with permission of Allergan, Inc.)

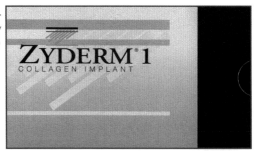

Figure 9-2. Zyderm 2® collagen implants are purified fibrillar suspensions of bovine collagen, 6.5% by weight. (Reprinted with permission of Allergan, Inc.)

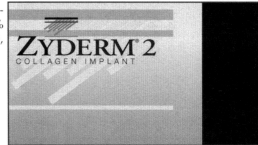

Figure 9-3. Zyplast® collagen implant contains 3.5% by weight bovine collagen, however, unlike Zyderm®, the collagen in Zyplast® is lightly cross-linked by the addition of 0.0075% glutaraldehyde. (Reprinted with permission of Allergan, Inc.)

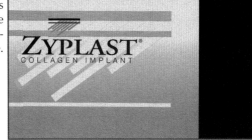

Zyderm 1 and 2 and Zyplast collagen implants are each sterile, purified fibrillar suspensions of bovine dermal collagen. Zyderm collagen implants consist of 95% to 98% type I collagen; the remainder is type III collagen.[22] These collagen proteins are suspended in phosphate-buffered physiologic saline containing 0.3% lidocaine. Zyderm 1 and Zyderm 2 collagen implants differ only in concentration. Zyderm 1 is 3.5% by weight bovine collagen, whereas Zyderm 2 is 6.5% by weight bovine collagen (Figures 9-1 and 9-2).

Zyplast bovine dermal collagen implants also contain 3.5% by weight bovine collagen; however, the collagen in Zyplast is lightly cross-linked by the addition of 0.0075% glutaraldehyde. Glutaraldehyde cross-links by producing covalent bridges between 10% of available lysine residues of the bovine collagen molecule. As a result, Zyplast is more resistant to proteolytic degradation and less immunogenic than Zyderm. The more substantive nature of Zyplast makes it applicable for deeper contour defects that are often unresponsive to Zyderm 1 or Zyderm 2 (Figure 9-3).[14]

When bovine sources of collagen are used as filler agents, the risk of transmissible disease must be considered. Both Zyderm and Zyplast are derived from the skin of a secluded American herd of Angus/Hereford cattle that has lived in the same location in California for 30 years, minimizing the possibility of contamination with the bovine spongiform encephalopathy prion.[23] In fact, there has never been a report of prion disease transmission with use of bovine collagen.

Both Zyderm and Zyplast are provided in preloaded syringes that must be stored at a low temperature (4°C) so that the dispersed fibrils remain fluid and small. This allows passage of the products through small-gauge needles. Once implanted, the human body temperature causes the collagen to undergo consolidation into a solid gel.[22] Following injection into the dermis, Zyderm and Zyplast are incorporated into the host tissue without discernible encapsulation and reproduce the texture, consistency, and structural integrity of the host tissue.[24]

Allergenicity and Contraindications

In addition to the theoretical concern of transmissible disease, there is also the concern for potential allergic reactions to bovine collagen. Individuals who have a history of an anaphylactic event or previous sensitivity to bovine collagen or a known dietary allergy to beef should also be excluded from testing and treatment. Because these products also contain lidocaine, patients with a known sensitivity to lidocaine should also be excluded.

For patients without a known history of sensitivity to bovine collagen, potential allergenicity to injectable bovine collagen must be determined by skin testing.[25] A positive reaction to skin testing is an absolute contraindication to treatment. A skin test syringe is provided by the manufacturer and contains 0.3 mL Zyderm 1. It is used to screen for allergies to both Zyderm and Zyplast therapy. Using only one-third of the test syringe's contents, the 0.1-mL dose should be administered (similar to a tuberculin skin test) into the dermis of the volar forearm. The site is then evaluated at 48 to 72 hours and again at 4 weeks.[25] A positive skin test is defined as swelling, induration, tenderness, or erythema that persists for 6 hours or longer within 4 weeks after the test implantation. Seventy percent of these reactions will become manifest in 48 to 72 hours, indicating a pre-existing allergy to bovine collagen. Since most reactions occur within 3 days of testing, it is recommended that the test site be evaluated at 48 to 72 hours and then again at 4 weeks. A positive skin test response has been estimated to occur in 3.0% to 3.5% of individuals undergoing first time skin testing (Figures 9-4 to 9-7).[23]

An additional 2% of patients develop an allergic reaction at the treatment site despite an initial negative skin test (Figure 9-8). Therefore, most authorities now recommend a second test as an additional precaution.[26,27] This second injection can be placed either in the contralateral forearm or in the periphery of the face (near the hairline). The second skin test is administered 4 weeks after initial testing, with treatment commencing 6 weeks after the first test was administered if both test sites show no evidence of reaction. Because the majority of treatment-associated hypersensitivity reactions occur shortly after the first treatment in patients who received only a single skin test, double testing is believed to greatly reduce the frequency of allergic reactions. Furthermore, treatment-associated hypersensitivity reactions that do occur after 2 negative skin test results tend to be milder, indicating that the most severely allergic patients have been excluded from collagen therapy. Single retesting of individuals who have not been treated for more than 1 year or who were successfully tested or treated elsewhere is strongly recommended.[1] In such cases, after retesting, a minimum of 2 weeks of observation is recommended before commencing with treatment.[1]

In addition to patients with a positive skin test, any patient currently on corticosteroid or immunosuppressive therapy (eg, prednisone) should be excluded from bovine collagen therapy. A history of autoimmune disease that includes but is not limited to rheumatoid arthritis, psoriatic arthritis, scleroderma (included CREST syndrome), systemic or discoid lupus erythematosus, or polymyositis represents a relative contraindication to bovine collagen therapy. The use of bovine collagen therapy in pregnant females and children has not been studied and is discouraged.

Figure 9-4. Collagen test kits consist of test syringes each containing 0.3 mL Zyderm 1®. (Reprinted with permission of Allergan, Inc.)

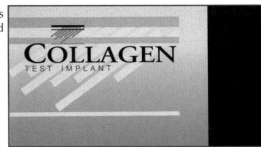

Figure 9-5. When skin testing, administer only one third of the test syringe's contents (0.1 mL) into the dermis of the volar forearm.

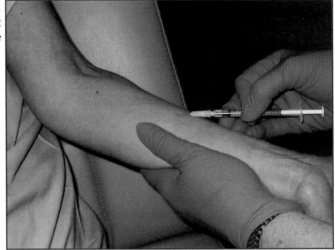

Figure 9-6. A negative skin test photographed at 72 hours. (Reprinted with permission of Allergan, Inc.)

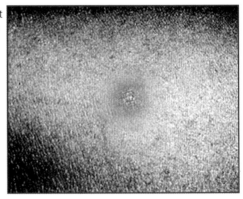

Since bovine collagen requires skin testing and has an increased allergic profile compared with human collagen, injection techniques and methods will be described for human collagen.

Human Collagen

In response to the antigenic limitations of bovine collagen, Inamed developed 2 cadaver-derived human collagen products, CosmoDerm® and CosmoPlast® (Allergan, Inc). They are the only FDA approved dermal fillers that contain bioengineered type I/type III human collagen, with phosphate-buffered saline and 0.3% lidocaine.[16] Unlike

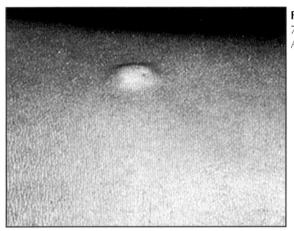

Figure 9-7. A positive skin test photographed at 72 hours. (Reprinted with permission of Allergan, Inc.)

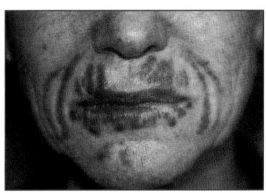

Figure 9-8. Collagen hypersensitivity reaction. (Courtesy of Leslie Baumann.)

bovine collagen, CosmoDerm and CosmoPlast do not require a skin test prior to clinical administration since the incidence of allergic reaction in controlled studies was 1.3%. This allows for same-day evaluation and treatment of rhytides, which is an advantage for both the physician and patient.

CosmoDerm is marketed in 2 forms, CosmoDerm 1 and CosmoDerm 2, and is analogous to Zyderm 1 and Zyderm 2 in terms of percent collagen and indicated usage. CosmoPlast is analogous to Zyplast collagen implant. Both CosmoDerm 1 and 2 and CosmoPlast contain collagen purified from human fibroblast cell cultures. The cell line used for collagen production is qualified by extensive testing for viruses, retroviruses, cell morphology, karyology, isoenzymes, and tumorigenicity.

Like Zyderm, CosmoDerm 1 and CosmoDerm 2 collagen implants are sterile devices composed of highly purified human-based collagen that is dispersed in phosphate-buffered physiological saline containing 0.3% lidocaine. CosmoDerm, like Zyderm, exists in a non–cross-linked form. CosmoDerm 2 collagen implant contains almost twice the collagen concentration of CosmoDerm 1 collagen implant. CosmoPlast collagen implant is also a highly purified human-based collagen that, like Zyplast, is cross-linked with glutaraldehyde and dispersed in phosphate-buffered physiological saline containing 0.3% lidocaine.

CosmoDerm 1 and 2 and CosmoPlast implants are supplied in individual sterile treatment syringes with needles and are packaged for single patient use. CosmoDerm and CosmoPlast implants should be stored at standard refrigerator temperatures (2°C to 10°C/36°F to 50°F).

Indications

CosmoDerm 1 and CosmoDerm 2 are designed for the correction of superficial facial wrinkles and should be injected as superficially as possible into the papillary dermis. CosmoDerm 1 is considered the most versatile of all forms of injectable collagen. It is effective in smoothing glabellar frown lines, horizontal forehead lines, marionette lines, perioral smile lines, crow's feet, and vertical lip lines. It is also effective in the treatment of certain types of shallow scars. CosmoDerm 1 contains approximately 30% to 35% collagen. The remainder of each syringe is saline and lidocaine hydrochloride, which disperses into soft tissue within 48 hours after injection, leaving only the collagen implant.[7]

CosmoDerm 2 contains approximately 60% to 70% collagen, which is nearly twice the amount of collagen contained in CosmoDerm 1. Indications for CosmoDerm 2 include horizontal forehead lines, glabellar lines, nasolabial lines, marionette lines, and shallow acne scars. It should not be used in the delicate eyelid skin or for treatment of radial lip lines, as lumping and whitish discoloration within the treated skin may occur because of its more viscous nature.

CosmoPlast was designed for placement into the middle to deep (reticular) dermis. It is used for more pronounced contour problems (such as deeper scars, lines, and furrows) and for areas where greater muscular activity is going to cause dissolution and breakdown of the compound (such as the lip). Because there have been case reports of vascular compromise within the glabellar area after injection with CosmoPlast, it is not recommended for treatment of glabellar frown lines.

Regardless of its source, correction in collagen replacement therapy is temporary at best and requires periodic reinjections to maintain desired results.[1] Correction is probably lost because the material is slowly displaced from its site of implantation within the dermis into the subcutaneous space.[22] Most patients require periodic touch-up treatment as early as 3 months after the initial injection.

Treatment Techniques

CosmoDerm collagen is implanted in the superficial dermis by serial punctures into the skin with a 30-gauge needle. The material is injected with the bevel directed up at a depth of approximately 1 mm so that the bevel of the needle is just visible beneath the surface of the skin. As a reference, the bevel of a standard 30-gauge needle is approximately 1 mm in diameter and serves as a useful guide for the proper depth of placement. CosmoDerm and CosmoPlast are also supplied with an adjustable depth gauge (ADG) needle. There is a circular plastic collar that is located next to the needle hub, which allows a protective guard to be advanced over the shaft of the needle. This ensures proper injection depth and placement of CosmoDerm or CosmoPlast within the superficial and mid dermal layers (Figure 9-9).

When implanting CosmoDerm 1, the syringe is held nearly parallel to the skin surface. While injecting, it is often helpful to stabilize the treatment area by holding the skin in the area being treated tautly between the thumb and forefinger of the noninjecting hand. Upon injecting, the material should flow evenly into the superficial dermis, causing a flat yellow blanching of the skin. A pronounced wheal should appear following blanching, indicating adequate over-correction. Each subsequent injection volume should be placed at the advancing edge of the previously injected quantity, generating a continuum of material that smoothly fills in the defect (Figure 9-10).

CosmoDerm 1 is the most sensitive technique, but also the most forgiving. Because it is not cross-linked, it flows easily within the dermis. When placed correctly, it will smoothly fill superficial defects. Although persistent beading and over-correction can be problematic with superficial placement of CosmoDerm 1 in the periocular and eyelid

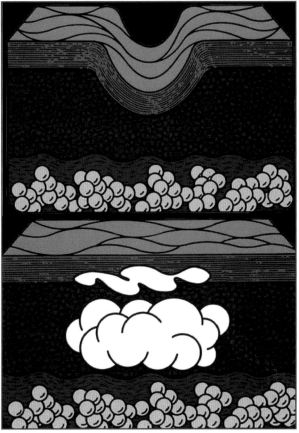

Figure 9-9. Proper depth placement of CosmoDerm® and CosmoPlast® collagen. CosmoDerm® collagen is deposited within the superficial papillary dermis at a depth of approximately 1 mm. CosmoPlast® collagen is injected deeper, within the mid-reticular dermis at a depth of approximately 2 mm. (Reprinted with permission of Allergan, Inc.)

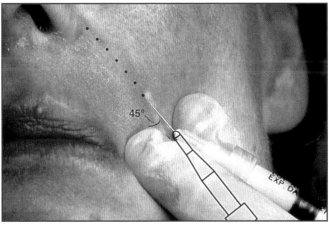

Figure 9-10. Treatment of nasolabial folds with CosmoPlast® collagen. (Reprinted with permission of Allergan, Inc.)

skin, beading is unlikely elsewhere. In general, up to 200% correction is indicated, except in the periorbital areas where correction should be limited to 100%.[16]

Techniques for injection with CosmoDerm 2 are almost identical to those outlined above for CosmoDerm 1. Like CosmoDerm 1, CosmoDerm 2 also contains non–cross-linked microfibrils and flows easily within the dermis. However, because of its greater collagen concentration, CosmoDerm 2 requires greater mechanical force to inject and it undergoes less condensation upon implantation.[7] With superficial placement of CosmoDerm 2, only modest over-correction is recommended to avoid persistent whiteness at the injection site. A slight degree of over-correction of only 110% to 120% should be sought when injecting CosmoDerm 2.

In the utilization of CosmoPlast, a 30-gauge needle is employed to place the material at the mid dermal level using a serial puncture technique. As mentioned previously, CosmoPlast is cross-linked and lacks microfibrils and undergoes little syneresis or condensation upon implantation. Therefore, it is more resistant to even flow within the dermis. CosmoPlast should be placed neither too superficially nor in the subdermal space.[16] Injection in the superficial dermis will result in persistent over-correction with beading and will not provide lasting correction in the subcutaneous layer. Ideally, it should be placed within the middle to deep reticular dermis (2 mm below the skin surface).[28] One hundred percent correction is recommended when using CosmoPlast.

Unlike the serial puncture technique that is utilized elsewhere for CosmoPlast, augmentation of the vermilion border of the lip is best accomplished with a linear threading technique. While some individuals advocate using a serial "pushing" approach in which the material is injected upon insertion of the needle, this can create lumping or beading in individuals who have fibrosis from previous dermal filler injections along the lip line. For this reason, it is best to consider a serial "pulling" technique in which a 30-gauge, 0.5-inch or 1-inch needle is inserted to its full extent and material is injected as the needle is withdrawn. The needle tract provides a potential space that will allow the material to flow into the vermilion border without associated beading issues. Augmentation of the vermilion border with CosmoPlast is a nice adjunct to volumetric augmentation of the lip with hyaluronic fillers, which is discussed in greater detail later in this chapter.

When injecting CosmoPlast, the syringe is held at a 45-degree to 90-degree angle. To achieve this angle, it may be helpful to rest the syringe over the finger or thumb of the noninjecting hand. The needle is injected with the bevel directed up and because of the greater depth of injection, the bevel is usually not visible beneath the skin. While implanting CosmoPlast, the resistance of the dermal matrix is felt against the injecting hand, and the plane of the injected site should elevate as the material is being placed. If a "pop" or sudden loss of resistance is felt while injecting CosmoPlast, this indicates that the needle has passed into the subdermal space. Should this occur, the needle should be withdrawn and then reinjected into the dermis. For CosmoPlast collagen, a delayed blanch is observed upon correction. If no blanching occurs, the placement of the needle may be too deep. Since over-correction is not recommended with CosmoPlast, no wheal should be raised. Although some advocate the practice of molding or massing CosmoPlast after implantation in order to avoid beading, others maintain that aggressive massage may result in the rapid loss of correction as the material is forced into the subdermal space.[11]

The simultaneous use of both CosmoDerm and CosmoPlast can often provide a superior result compared to single agent therapy, both in regard to cosmetic result and in persistence of improvement. For example, increased longevity of correction and improved aesthetic results can often be achieved by the layering technique wherein CosmoDerm 2 is immediately implanted over CosmoPlast injection sites. This is especially true in the treatment of deep nasolabial lines/folds and marionette lines.

Correction with CosmoDerm and CosmoPlast is temporary and requires periodic reinjections to maintain desired results. Correction is probably lost because the material is slowly displaced from its site of implantation within the dermis into the subcutaneous space. For all etiologies, 30% of individuals who have undergone collagen injections report persistent correction at 18 months post-treatment. However, the majority (70%) require touch-up treatments at intervals of 3 to 12 months. Areas under the greatest stress such as the lips require more frequent maintenance injections, while glabellar frown lines and acne scars appear to retain correction the longest.[16] Patients should expect periodic touch-ups every 3 to 4 months.

Allergenicity and Complications

Manufacturers suggest that CosmoDerm and CosmoPlast should not be used in patients with severe allergies manifested by a history of anaphylaxis. All dermal filler agents must also be used with caution in patients who are atopic or who have a history of multiple allergies. The safety of use of CosmoDerm and CosmoPlast in patients with a known hypersensitivity to bovine collagen has not yet been determined.

In a study to evaluate sensitization to CosmoDerm and CosmoPlast, 428 patients had CosmoDerm 1 injected intradermally into the volar forearm and were then followed for 2 months. Reported adverse events included cold and flu-like symptoms, urinary tract infection, bronchitis, Strep throat, sinus infection, ear infection, fever, insomnia, sore throat, high-blood pressure, acid dyspepsia or reflux, back ache, and muscle spasm.[28]

Of note, one subject in this study reported redness and pain at 1 week after injection. This was confirmed as localized redness, tenderness, induration, and edema at the injection site. These symptoms spontaneously resolved after 10 days without treatment or sequelae. The absence of an antibody response against CosmoDerm and histopathological examination of a biopsy of the injection site suggested that the injection site reaction was not immunologically related to CosmoDerm injection.[28]

HYALURONIC ACID DERIVATIVES

The demand for HA fillers is based on the fact that they are less likely to cause an allergic reaction and tend to last up to 3 to 6 months longer than collagen-based products.[29,30] Global sales have grown from $40 million in 2004 to over $300 million in 2005. HA derivatives vary between the source of HA (avian or bacterial), concentration of HA, particle size, whether or not the HA is cross-linked, the type of cross-linking agent used, and viscosity.[31]

HA is a basic building block of the dermis. It is a naturally occurring glycosaminoglycan that is a major component of all connective tissue. It exhibits no species or tissue specificity, as the chemical structure of this polysaccharide is uniform throughout nature. There is no potential for immunologic reactions to HA in humans. HA molecules in the skin bind water and create volume. HA is a monomer composed of sodium glucuronate combined with N-actyl glucosamine. The HA is manufactured as a polymer that is composed of multiple monomers bound together like a string of beads. In its non–cross-linked form, HA is essentially a liquid since the molecules are suspended individually in solution. Cross-linking HA increases the cohesiveness of the product and transforms its liquid configuration into a gel. The hardness of the gel relates to the amount of cross-linking that is present in commercially available HA compounds. Other parameters that affect hardness include the concentration of HA as well as the sizing of the gel particles within the compound. To reduce gel hardness parameters for a given compound, uncross-linked HA is typically added to cross-linked HA to thin the agent and increase flow. This can also be accomplished by adding smaller HA gel particles.

The amount of HA in the skin decreases with age, and its loss results in reduced dermal hydration and increased skin wrinkling/folding. Because of the very low potential for immunologic reactions to HA (a risk of 1 out of 2000), it has become an attractive alternative to collagen replacement therapy throughout Canada and Europe. Several of these products are now available in the United States and more products are in the final stages of FDA trials.

Figure 9-11. Restylane.

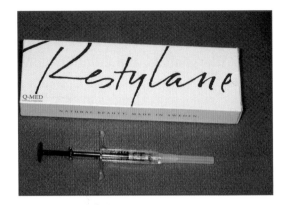

Figure 9-12. Intended areas of placement for hyaluronic derivatives.

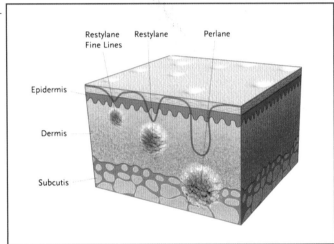

Restylane

Restylane® (Q-Med, Uppsala, Sweden) (Figure 9-11) is a HA soft tissue filler that is made of HA biosynthetically produced through a bacterial fermentation process. It has led to a resurgence in the use of dermal filler agents and currently has dominant market share in the United States where it is marketed by Medicis Aesthetics, Inc of Scottsdale, Ariz. Since it is produced by bacterial fermentation in the lab, Restylane is referred to as a NASHA compound. It is minimally cross-linked or stabilized with 1,4-butane-diol diglycidyl ether (BDDE).[32] Upon injection into tissue, the NASHA gel dissipates, binds water, and increases in volume. The volume is maintained until the HA is degraded and disappears completely over time.

Three forms of the product are currently available: Restylane Touch® also marketed as Restylane Fine Lines®, Restylane, and Perlane®. Currently, only Restylane and Perlane are FDA approved for aesthetic use in the United States but approval for Restylane Touch is expected in 2007. Each compound was originally designed to be injected into different layers of the skin (Figure 9-12). In addition to these regions, Perlane has been found to be useful in facial contouring and may be injected below the dermis as well as in the preperiosteal plane to correct deeper volume deficits. The physical difference between the products is the size of the gel particle.

Restylane Touch has 500,000 gel particles per mL and is used for fine superficial wrinkles. Restylane has 100,000 gel particles per mL and is used for larger wrinkles (eg,

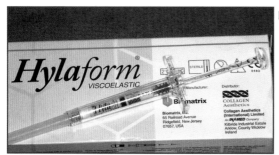

Figure 9-13. Hylaform.

glabellar furrows, nasolabial lines, lip augmentation) (see Figure 9-11). Perlane (10,000 gel particles per mL) is used for deeper folds (nasolabial) and volume augmentation (lips). The HA concentration of Restylane is 20 mg/mL. Eighty percent of this exists in the cross-linked form while 20% is uncross-linked to increase flow tendencies. The products are designed to last between 6 and 8 months. Since there is no species or tissue specificity, there is very limited potential for immunologic reactions to the HA. Skin testing is therefore not required. Local injection-related reactions occasionally occur and may include transient erythema, pain, itching, and tenderness.[33]

Hylaform

Hylaform® and Hylaform Plus® (Inamed) (Figure 9-13) are HA soft tissue fillers similar to Restylane. The concentration of HA is 6 mg/mL and is extracted from rooster combs.[34] To date, there have been no reported instances of immunologic reactions to any residual avian products, but the trend has been to avoid animal products in lieu of products produced by bacterial fermentation.[13] Hylaform is roughly equivalent to Restylane and is used in similar wrinkle areas (glabella, nasolabial folds, marionette lines, lip augmentation, etc). Like Restylane, Hylaform also comes in a thicker version (Hylaform Plus). The duration of effect is slightly less than Restylane (6 months versus 6 to 8 months) but is individually dependant. While no skin test is required for either product, the trend among physicians is to avoid animal-sourced HA.[35]

Captique

To circumvent the aversion to animal-based HA products, Inamed recently launched Captique® (Figure 9-14), which is a NASHA compound with a concentration of 5.5 mg/mL. It is indicated for the correction of moderate to severe lines with a duration of approximately 6 months. At the time of publication, it has not significantly penetrated the market since Restylane is so well established among practitioners.

Juvéderm

Juvéderm™ is an export from France that has been used for the past several years.[36] Juvéderm is a product of LEA Derm Laboratories, a subsidiary of Corneal Group (Paris, France) and is also a HA that is of nonanimal origin that will be exclusively marketed in the United States, Canada, and Australia by Allergan Inc. Allergan has nonexclusive rights in France, Spain, the United Kingdom, Italy, Germany, and Switzerland where it will be established with a new brand name: Hydra Fill® 1, 2, and 3. Juvéderm is a patented single-phase cross-linked BDDE HA that is phosphate buffered to a pH of 6.5 to 7.3.[36] It has been recently FDA approved in the United States in 2 forms: Juvéderm 24™, which will be marketed in the United States as Juvéderm Ultra™, and Juvéderm 24 HV™, which

Figure 9-14. Captique.

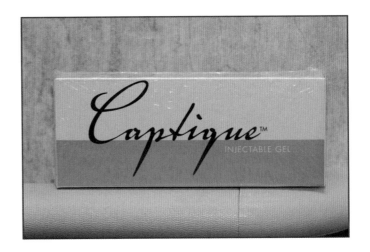

will be marketed in the United States as Juvéderm Ultra Plus™. All of these agents are indicated for lip augmentation, reduction of nasolabial folds, and subdermal facial sculpting. The duration of action is 6 to 9 months but like the other HA products is individually dependant. All of these agents do not require a skin test, are biocompatible, and have the highest concentration of HA available today (24 mg/mL of HA). While 90% of the HA is in its cross-linked form, 10% of it is not cross-linked to facilitate smoothness and consistency. The difference between Juvéderm Ultra and Juvéderm Ultra Plus relates to the percentage of cross-linking between the HA molecules. Juvéderm Ultra has 6% cross-linking, which means that for every 100 HA monomers, 6 of them are cross-linked to an adjacent HA molecule. In contrast, Juvéderm Ultra Plus has 8% cross-linking, which increases the thickness of the compound. The major difference between Juvéderm, Restylane, and other NASHA forms of HA relates to variable particle sizing. For example, Restylane is composed of equal-sized gel particles with approximately 100,000 gel particles per mL. In contrast, Juvéderm is composed of a variety of gel particle sizes. Some of these particles are smaller than those found in Restylane while some are substantially larger. This particle size heterogeneity provides a smoother consistency to the product, which reduces the percentage of uncross-linked HA that is needed to reduce gel hardness and improve injection flow. As such, Restylane utilizes 20% uncross-linked HA while Juvéderm is able to maintain good flow consistency with 10% cross-linked HA.

In summary, Juvéderm has the highest total concentration of HA as well as the highest concentration of cross-linked HA when compared to all other NASHA fillers. Its variable particle sizing also contributes to its flow parameters, which allow a greater percentage of cross-linked HA to be used with a smaller percentage of uncross-linked HA.

In addition, experienced injectors feel that Juvéderm is easy to work with and has a pliable feel and a slightly longer duration of effect than other agents on the market (Leslie Baumann, oral communication, March 2005).

Adverse Reactions

Some common injection-related reactions may occur following the injection of HA fillers. They include erythema, swelling, pain, itching, bruising, and tenderness at the implant site. These reactions have generally been described as mild to moderate and typically resolve spontaneously a few days after injection.

Adverse treatment responses to HA fillers can be divided into nonhypersensitive and hypersensitive reactions. The most common nonhypersensitive reactions are transient

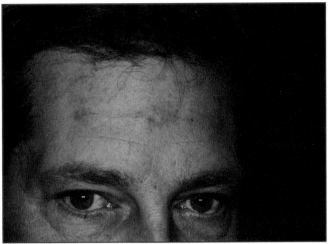

Figure 9-15. Six months post-Restylane injection, the patient returned with prominent red lines along the horizontal forehead.

and mild and include bruising, reactivation of herpetic eruptions, and localized bacterial infection.[37] Some areas (such as compressed scars) resist precise placement of the material, resulting in a slight elevation beside the actual defect.[33]

More serious nonhypersensitive reactions include vascular interruption at the treatment site with subsequent localized tissue necrosis and intravascular injection of collagen, causing distal embolic events.[38] Vascular interruption caused by injection is much more likely to occur with more viscous agents (eg, Perlane and Juvéderm Ultra Plus) because it is intended to be injected deeper near the vascular supply of the dermis and because it is slower to undergo syneresis after injection. The incidence of vascular occlusion is reportedly approximately 0.09% of all treated patients. Because 56% of all reported necrotic events occur in the glabellar area, physicians are cautioned against using CosmoPlast and Perlane at this site. The basis for the increased incidence in the glabellar area has been shown to be due to a lack of collateral circulation in this area when branches of the supratrochlear artery are temporarily occluded.[39]

Reactions thought to be of a hypersensitive nature have been reported in about 1 in every 2000 treated patients. Granuloma or abscess formation, localized necrosis, and urticaria have been reported in rare instances (Figure 9-15). Tissue necrosis results in scab formation followed by sloughing of the tissue at the treatment site, which results in a shallow scar. If the practitioner notes severe blanching of the area and the patient complains of pain upon injection, the injection should immediately be stopped because local necrosis has possibly occurred. The value of massage, warm compresses, or nitroglycerin gel in this situation is, as yet, unsubstantiated, but any or all these therapies may be utilized in an attempt to limit the loss of tissue. If tissue necrosis occurs, maintain good wound care as the tissue sloughs in order to prevent infection and to allow healing to occur.

Puragen

Puragen™ and Puragen Plus™ (Mentor Corp, Santa Barbara, Calif) are the first HA-based injectables to utilize a new form of crosslinking called DXL. This patented process double cross-links hyaluron molecules, providing greater resistance to degradation than single cross-linked HA fillers. DXL technology is a process that stabilizes HA molecules with 2 separate types of bonds. DXL uses 1,2,7,8-diepoxyoctane to create both ether and ester bonds. This molecular configuration slows the degradation rate of the compound by reducing the rate of diffusion of the hyaluronidase enzyme into the matrix. Theoretically,

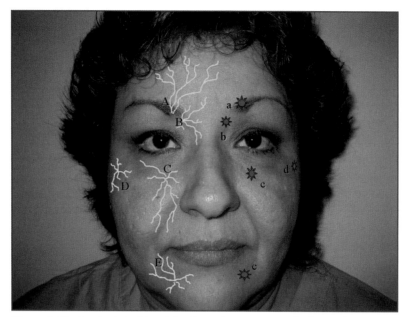

Figure 9-16. On the left side of the face, the images marked in yellow correspond to the major branches of the sensory nerves of the face: (A) supraorbital bundle; (B) supratrochlear and infra-trochlear bundle; (C) infraorbital bundle; (D) zygomaticofacial bundle; and (E) submental bundle. On the right side of the face, points (a) through (e) correspond to the location of appropriate injection to provide anesthesia of these major nerve roots.

Puragen should have the benefits of smaller particle agents (ie, ease of injection and broader applications) with the benefit of larger particle resilience, which should extend the duration of clinical effect. As such, one product will be able to provide the benefits that previously required multiple agents with varying particle size. Puragen is produced in the lab as a bacterial fermentation product and is not derived from animal sources, reducing allergic reaction concerns.

Puragen Plus with DXL technology is a new agent that is expected to be released in 2007 and will include lidocaine similar to collagen filler agents. The advantage of a built-in anesthetic is appealing since HA injections can be painful and require regional nerve blocks for anesthesia. The double cross-linking of the HA molecule in Puragen provides increased molecular stability that permits the incorporation of lidocaine, which will increase both patient satisfaction and comfort.

Pretreatment Anesthesia

Even when an agent is premixed with lidocaine, injection of all filler agents can be painful, which may ultimately affect the patient's motivation for repeat treatments. The use of a local, regional, and/or topical anesthesia, when applicable, may improve patient discomfort. Regional nerve blocks provide adequate anesthesia without distorting the tissues that are to be augmented (Figure 9-16 and Table 9-2). This is usually the best anesthesia approach when injecting HA fillers. A mixture of lidocaine 1% with 1:100,000 dilution of epinephrine is usually adequate. It is also helpful to coadminister topical anesthesia with regional nerve blocks to augment the anesthetic effect. Local injection of anesthesia is also

Table 9-2

General Guide for Anesthetic/Nerve Blocks for Particular Facial Regions

Target Lesion Defect	Regional/Local Anesthetic
Glabellar frown lines (and horizontal furrows at root of nose/overlying procerus muscle	Infratrochlear, supratrochlear and supraorbital, and frontolacrimal nerve blocks
Horizontal forehead furrow	Frontolacrimal nerve block
Lateral canthal rhytides	Transconjunctival/local
Nasolabial folds	Infraorbital nerve black (transcutaneous or trans-buccal
Lip augmentation	Transbuccal/local
Marionette lines	Transbuccal (lower gingival sulcus)
Perioral rhytides (vertical)	Transbuccal

helpful in achieving anesthetic effect, but the infiltration of the anesthetic tends to distort the areas intended for augmentation. One advantage, however, is local vasoconstriction, which may lead to less bruising and swelling and may serve to minimize the risk of inadvertent intravascular injection. To minimize tissue distortion, injections may be performed from within the oral cavity similar to gingival dental nerve blocks (Figure 9-17).

Topical anesthesia may be applied to the area prior to injection to reduce discomfort. I have found that topical CaineTips® (J. Morita USA, Inc, Irvine, Calif) work well to diminish local anesthetic injection discomfort of the oral mucosa. The applicator is applied to the area for 15 to 30 seconds prior to the injection and comes in a variety of flavors (Figure 9-18). A combination of topical oral mucosal anesthesia combined with regional nerve blocks and local infiltration is my current preferred anesthesia technique.

EMLA cream (2.5% lidocaine and 2.5% prilocaine), betacaine, and similar topical anesthetic agents can be useful before injection. While topical anesthetics produce adequate anesthesia to reduce the discomfort associated with percutaneous needle penetrations, they do not work well to reduce the pain associated with instillation of HA fillers from tissue expansion. For maximum effectiveness, topical anesthetics must be applied at least 30 minutes to 1 hour before treatment (Figure 9-19).[40]

Pretreatment Preparation

The use of drugs that reduce coagulation such as aspirin and NSAIDs may result in increased bruising or bleeding at the injection sites. Therefore, treatment with any dermal filler agent should be delayed until these agents have been discontinued for at least 1 week. Active inflammatory skin conditions (eruptions such as cysts, pimples, rashes, or hives) or infections also require that treatment be postponed until the condition has been controlled.[28]

Proper informed consent and pretreatment photographic documentation is of paramount importance. Patients should remove any make-up from the face and wash it with mild soap and water on the day of treatment. The patient should be placed in an upright position in a comfortable chair. Overhead lighting should be used so that contour deficiencies are accentuated. Loupe magnification is helpful and often essential for correct depth of placement. The skin in the area to be treated should be prepped with alcohol or a

Figure 9-17. A gingival nerve block is an excellent technique to provide anesthesia for the correction of nasolabial folds and lip augmentation. The needle is inserted above the canine tooth in the gingival sulcus and directed below the inferior orbital rim. Typically 1 cc to 2 cc of anesthesia is adequate.

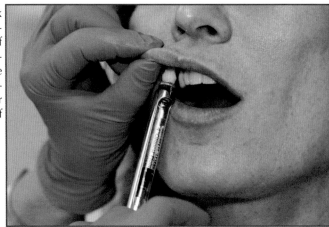

Figure 9-18. (A) To reduce the discomfort of a gingival injection, the gingival sulcus may be anesthetized with a topical CaineTip. (B) A topical CaineTip is pre-filled with a 20% benzocaine solution.

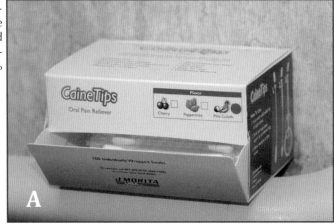

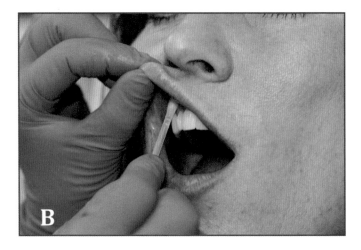

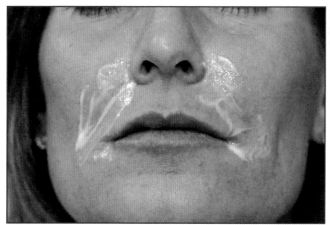

Figure 9-19. Topical anesthetics should be applied 30 minutes prior to injection.

similar antiseptic. Some physicians prefer prepping the skin with a povidone-iodine solution. Many physicians have found it helpful to outline the scar or wrinkle to be treated with a surgical marking pen. When augmenting multiple sites, concentrate on getting full correction at one site before treating other sites.

CosmoDerm and CosmoPlast must be stored at +2°C to 10°C until time of injection. The material should not be frozen. The product may be stored for use until its marked date of expiration. The pre-filled syringes are designed for 1-time, single patient use. The collagen-filled syringe should be removed from the refrigerator at least 30 minutes before use. A 30-gauge needle is then firmly affixed to the Luer-lock end of the syringe. A small test amount should be injected into the needle, and collagen should be seen exiting the lumen of the needle. This ensures normal syringe and needle function and allows the physician to evaluate the level of resistance prior to injection within the dermis.

HA fillers may be stored between 2°C and 25°C (either refrigerated or at room temperature). Most products have a shelf life of 12 to 18 months. Like collagen, the material should not be placed in a freezer. A 30-gauge needle is typically used for thinner products like Restylane and Juvéderm Ultra, while a 27-gauge needle is recommended for thicker agents like Perlane and Juvéderm Ultra Plus. The HA-filled syringe should be allowed to attain room temperature prior to injection.

Injection Techniques and Tips

Selection of the appropriate injectable implant often depends on the depth of the wrinkle and the intended site of injection of the filler. Some fillers are more viscous and require placement in the subcutaneous space, while others are more fluid and can be injected more superficially within the dermis. Fine, superficial rhytides respond best to fillers injected in the superficial dermis. Deeper, more substantial wrinkles often have a subcutaneous component and are best approached from the deeper dermis.[4] Furthermore, a wrinkle may have both a superficial and deep component, and both of these components may need to be addressed in order to obtain optimal treatment results.[5] Injection technique is believed to be the single most important factor in the successful application of collagen and HA implants. The ability to properly implant each agent requires a learning curve, and proper placement of the implant within the tissue will improve with experience.

It has been the authors' experience with temporary biodegradable filler agents that HA compounds are superior to collagen for the treatment of nasolabial folds, melomental folds, and lip volume augmentation. At present, the lower viscosity agents like Restylane Touch/Fine Lines, Hylaform Fine Lines® (Inamed), and Juvéderm 18™ are not FDA approved. For this reason, injection techniques for transverse forehead lines, periocular lines, crow's feet, and vertical lip lines are described using CosmoDerm 1. The lower viscosity HA compounds will likely replace CosmoDerm 1 for this indication once they are approved for use in the United States. Similarly, the higher viscosity HA compounds like Perlane and Juvéderm Ultra Plus will eventually replace CosmoPlast and Zyplast for filling in deeper lines and lip augmentation. It has been the authors' experience that lip augmentation is best accomplished with a combination of human collagen and HA fillers. The lidocaine present in CosmoPlast provides excellent supplemental anesthesia for the subsequent administration of HA compounds. Using this approach, the vermilion border is first defined with CosmoPlast while HA fillers are subsequently employed to augment lip volume.

The basic principles for injecting HA products are similar to the injection of collagen products. Unlike collagen products, which are best administered through a serial puncture technique, HA compounds are usually administered through a linear threading technique. All of the HA fillers are supplied as clear, transparent gels packaged in a disposable syringe

The amount supplied per syringe varies slightly as do the costs. In general, a 1-cc syringe of Restylane or Hylaform or a 0.8-cc syringe of Juvéderm will provide reasonable augmentation for a single (unilateral) nasolabial fold. One to 2 syringes may be required for lip augmentation and treatment of the lateral oral commisure. Traditionally, it has been felt that dermal filler agents need to be injected within the dermis. The less viscous fine line products (Restylane Fine Lines, Hylaform Fine Lines, Juvéderm 18) are injected in the upper dermis, the standard product (Restylane, Juvéderm 18) in the mid dermis, while the thicker products (Perlane, Juvéderm Ultra Plus) are placed in the deeper dermis.

A new trend in HA fillers has been to inject the fillers into the deeper dermis or subdermal plane to avoid exposure. In fact, treatment of the tear trough is now commonly performed as a facial sculpting procedure with Perlane and Juvéderm Ultra Plus in the preperiosteal plane. This is done to avoid rapid dissolution of the product, which would be experienced if the filler was injected into the orbicularis muscle, which has significant blood flow.

As mentioned previously, a linear threading technique is typically employed to inject HA fillers unlike collagen compounds, which are best injected with the serial puncture approach. Unlike serial puncture technique in which material is administered through multiple small injections that are typically made perpendicular to the line or wrinkle, linear threading typically involves administration of material along the axis of the line or wrinkle. Injection of the material is performed while inserting the needle or during its withdrawal. The needle is then placed further up or down the line and the injection is repeated in a similar fashion. With the bevel of the needle just visible beneath the skin, the needle is advanced to the leading edge of the line to be treated and the injection is made with constant pressure on the syringe plunger as the needle is withdrawn. The needle is then re-entered further down the line or fold in a similar fashion.

A standard 30-gauge needle permits smooth injection of Restylane, Captique, and Juvéderm, while thicker agents like Perlane or Juvéderm Ultra Plus require a 27-gauge needle (please see the DVD accompanying this text). There are 2 methods of linear threading that are frequently employed. One is referred to as the "linear pushing" technique while the other is referred to as the "linear pulling" technique. With "linear pushing," material is injected while the needle is inserted into the dermal or subdermal plane. While some individuals prefer this approach, proponents of the "linear pulling"

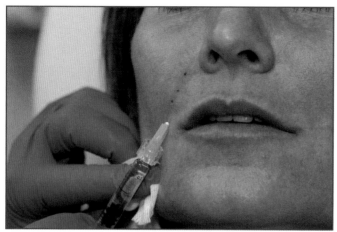

Figure 9-20. Linear threading injection techniqe for the treatment of nasolabial folds with HA.

technique note that a "pushing" approach can cause lumpiness or beading of the material in individuals who have undergone previous injections due to scar planes that have formed within the area of injection. The advantage of a "linear pulling" technique for individuals who have had dermal filler agents in the past is that the needle tract provides a potential space that allows more uniform expansion of the dermis and subdermal tissue (Figure 9-20). At present, there is no consensus to which approach is superior. Most injectors appear to favor either approach after they have obtained significant clinical experience injecting a variety of filler agents.

Successive threads may be laid down above, below, and beside the previous injections until the entire wrinkle or fold has been treated. If there are small depressions between the linear threads, isolated serial puncture injections may then be employed to fill in the gaps. Unlike collagen injections, which require over-correction to attain a desirable outcome (see Treatment Techniques on p. 112), HA fillers are used to smooth the wrinkle out as much as possible but not to over-correct the area. Once the products are injected, the material may be gently massaged along the line of injection to ensure the material is smooth. Each patient should be checked in 2 to 4 weeks for the adequacy of volume replacement. Some will require additional tissue augmentation for the desired effect.

Treatment of Prominent Nasolabial Folds

When treating nasolabial folds, experienced practitioners in the United States prefer to use Restylane, Perlane, Captique, Juvéderm Ultra, and/or Juvéderm Ultra Plus alone or in combination. Once the lower viscosity agents like Restylane Touch/Fine Lines and Juvéderm 18 become FDA approved in the United States, treatment with a combination of these HA filler agents will likely become the preferred treatment method. A linear "pulling" or "pushing" threading technique is recommended to ensure proper placement within the dermis or in the subdermal plane (see Figure 9-20).

It is also beneficial to mark the area that is to be treated. Water soluble markers work well for this purpose because they will not tattoo the skin if an injection is inadvertently placed through the area that has been marked. In my practice, I use Crayola (Binney & Smith Inc, Easton, Pa) water-soluble markers since they come in a variety of colors and can be used to indicate HA injection sites in one color and CosmoDerm 1 injections in a different color. Topical anesthesia using betacaine or EMLA may be applied to the region 20 to 30 minutes prior to injection. Since this area is also rather sensitive, a regional nerve

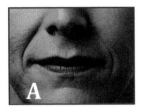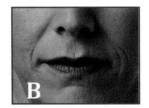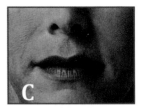

Figure 9-21. Prominent nasolabial folds (A) before treatment; (B) partial correction; (C) full correction with CosmoPlast®. (Reprinted with permission of Allergan, Inc.)

block provides optimal anesthesia and may be performed with a gingival dental block to inactivate the maxillary nerve (see Figure 9-16), or gingival sulcus anesthesia lateral to the nasal alar cartilage may also be employed (see Figure 9-17).

The HA filler should be deposited along the medial aspect of the nasolabial fold to flatten and efface the depression. The first injection is initiated approximately 1 cm to 2 cm below the lateral aspect of the nasal ala to place the HA filler into the upper end of the furrow at the lateral aspect of the nasal ala. A triangular fanning approach may be employed to fill a triangular depression inferolateral to the nasal alar cartilage. This can be further augmented by placing a vertical thread perpendicular to the previous injections to provide additional fill (please see the DVD accompanying this text).

Once the entire nasolabial fold has been treated, the HA filler may be massaged along either side of the injection pathway for more even distribution. Any gaps or depressions along the line may be treated with a serial puncture technique. If a fine line persists after augmentation with Restylane, consider a second layer of injection with CosmoDerm 1. When layering with CosmoDerm, a serial puncture technique should be used as described previously to deposit the material at a depth of 1 mm (Figures 9-20 and 9-21).

Treatment of Marionette or Melomental Lines

HA fillers like Restylane, Hylaform, Captique, or Juvéderm Ultra are recommended when treating prominent lines of the oral commissures using a linear "pulling" approach. The HA filler is injected once the tip of the needle has been advanced from the lateral aspect of the line to the edge of the vermilion border of the lip with a linear threading technique. The angle of the needle with respect to the skin surface is relatively flat (15 degrees to 30 degrees) and the skin should be stabilized on either side of the line with the noninjecting (nondominant) hand (Figure 9-22).

Manual massage may be helpful to smooth out any irregularities along the path of the injection. Digital massage may be performed with 1 finger in the mouth and another externally or with both fingers externally along the line of injection. If a fine line persists after augmentation with HA fillers, it can be softened by layering either CosmoDerm 1 or a lower viscosity HA filler agent more superficially into the dermis (typically 1 mm below the skin surface) (Figures 9-23 and 9-24).

Correction of Periocular Lines (Crow's Feet)

For those just beginning dermal filler injections, correction of periocular lines should be confined to the tissue outside of the orbital rim. Correction of periocular lines within the boundaries of the orbital rim is considered a more advanced technique and may result in a lumpy and unpleasant appearance. It is best to initiate treatments in this area outside of the orbital rim and extend treatment to involve the fine lines of the preseptal and

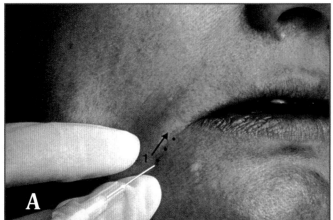

Figure 9-22. "Triangle" injection pattern for correction of melomental folds. (Reprinted with permission of Allergan, Inc.)

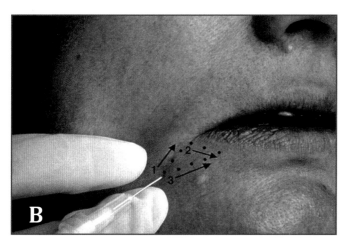

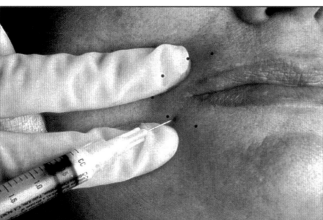

Figure 9-23. "Horseshoe" injection pattern for correction of melomental folds. (Reprinted with permission of Allergan, Inc.)

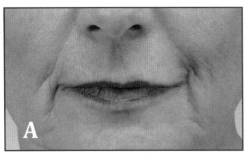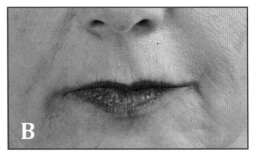

Figure 9-24. "Marionette" lines or melomental folds (A) before and (B) after augmentation with CosmoPlast®. (Reprinted with permission of Allergan, Inc.)

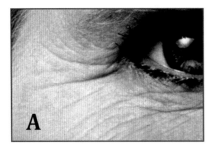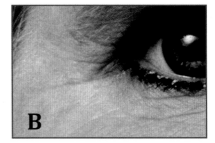

Figure 9-25. "Crow's feet" (A) before and (B) after augmentation with CosmoDerm® 1. (Reprinted with permission of Allergan, Inc.)

preorbital orbicularis muscle as you become more experienced with CosmoDerm injections. CosmoDerm 1 is recommended when treating periocular rhytides (Figure 9-25). When lower viscosity agents like Restylane Fine Lines and Juvederm 18 are FDA-approved, they will likely replace CosmoDerm injections. When injecting CosmoDerm 1, a serial puncture technique is enlisted and the needle is inserted at a angle of approximately 15 degrees to 30 degrees from the surface of the skin (Figure 9-26). While some injectors prefer to inject along the axis of the line or wrinkle, other individuals prefer injecting perpendicular to the axis of the line. With this approach, the needle is inserted along the lateral aspect of the line and the filler is injected underneath the linear depression to elevate the line. The needle is injected to a depth of less than 1 mm. CosmoDerm 1 comes with an ADG needle, which allows you to accurately determine the depth of injection. Typically a depth of 1 mm is utilized to correct "crow's feet" lines; inject to the point of blanching, but do not raise a wheal. Correct up to only 100% during any given treatment session. For complete correction, multiple light treatments at 1-week intervals may be necessary. If the crow's feet are not over-corrected, the final result can be very satisfying.

Correction of Nasal Tear Trough Deformities

There is a great deal of excitement regarding the utilization of HA fillers to diminish the appearance of nasal tear trough deformities. Experience with collagen injections has noted that subdermal injections result in rapid resorption and loss of treatment effect. Numerous investigators, however, are now injecting HA fillers in the subdermal plane to perform facial contouring and alleviate volume deficits like the tear trough deformity. A tear trough deformity is a linear depression that exists between the nasalis muscle and orbicularis muscle. As the malar fat pad descends, this indentation becomes more noticeable with time and is more common in thinner individuals who have less facial fat.

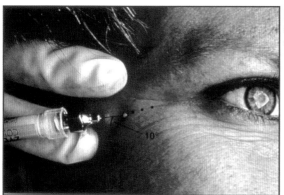

Figure 9-26. Injection technique for treating crow's feet with CosmoDerm 1®. (Reprinted with permission of Allergan, Inc.)

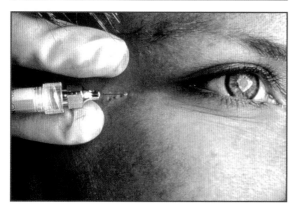

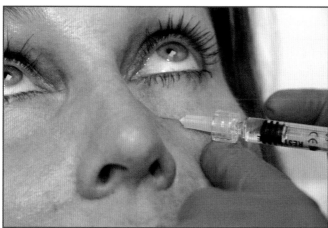

Figure 9-27. Correction of nasal tear trough deformity by injecting Juvéderm Ultra Plus™ in the preperiosteal plane (below the orbicularis oculi muscle).

At present, most authorities recommend injection of HA fillers for this purpose in a preperiosteal plane below the orbicularis and nasalis muscles. It is felt that the vascularity of these muscles will increase dissolution and degradation of the HA. Injection below the muscle, theoretically, should increase the longevity of the material since there is less muscular activity and blood flow within the preperiosteal plane (Figure 9-27).

For this purpose, thicker compounds such as Juvéderm Ultra Plus and Perlane are recommended. Lower density agents may also be used, but their longevity may not be as significant as the denser compounds that have a greater percentage of cross-linking and/or larger particle size. To perform the injections with Juvéderm Ultra Plus, the supplied needle is recommended. This needle is unique in that it has a 30-gauge outer diameter with a 27-gauge inner bore diameter. This allows Juvéderm Ultra Plus to be injected without the potential for shearing of the HA, which could break the larger particles into smaller pieces and reduce its longevity. The needle is inserted into the nasal aspect of the defect and HA is injected above but not in the periosteal plane.

Once the medial aspect of the tear trough deformity has been filled, the needle is withdrawn and inserted inferotemporally to fill the central portion of the defect. The lateral aspect of the defect is then filled with additional compound. Typically, 1 syringe or 0.8 mL of Juvéderm Ultra Plus or a 1-cc syringe of Perlane would be sufficient to correct one side of this volume deficiency.

Complications

Care should be taken to avoid injecting into the periosteum as this will cause significant discomfort. The angular artery is also located in the tear trough region. To avoid inadvertent injection of filler into the angular artery and potential embolization, it is reasonable to pull back on the syringe and see if any blood enters the syringe prior to injecting fillers into the medial aspect of the tear trough. If blood is encountered, the needle is withdrawn and pressure is applied. If frank blanching of the region is seen to occur, topical nitro paste may be administered to the region. The injector should make sure that nitro paste is administered with a gloved hand to avoid a vasodilatory headache and the patient should be advised that he or she will likely develop a headache secondary to administration of the nitro paste. This should, however, increase blood flow to the area. Since the angular artery is not an end artery, ischemic necrosis is not typically a concern. Given the relatively large diameter of the vessel and the fact that it has direct communication with the central nervous system, embolization of material into the central nervous system is a potential risk, albeit, a rather low risk. Withdrawing the needle prior to injection should reduce this risk significantly and potentially avoid this complication.

Correction of Glabellar Frown Lines

HA fillers like Restylane, Captique, or Juvéderm Ultra are recommended when treating glabellar frown lines (Figure 9-28). Avoid CosmoPlast, Perlane, or Juvéderm Ultra Plus because they carry an increased risk of disruption of the vascular supply in the glabellar skin due to their increased viscosity. Regional anesthesia may be performed with topical EMLA or a supratrochlear nerve block (see Figure 9-16).

The HA fillers should be injected directly into the line at a depth of 2 mm to 3 mm. A linear threading technique is utilized while the patient is placed in a slightly supine position in a clinical examination chair (see Figure 4-6). The needle is inserted at the inferior edge of the line above the orbital rim and directed toward the superior aspect of the vertical frown line. The filler agent is injected while the needle is withdrawn in a linear threading fashion (Figure 9-29).

If the implant extrudes upon injection into the thick glabellar skin, reposition the needle to a depth of 3 mm. If it continues to extrude, do not remove the needle; instead rotate it 1-quarter turn and continue to inject at a depth of 3 mm.

Correction of Horizontal Forehead Lines

Satisfactory treatment of horizontal forehead lines is difficult. The forehead skin is under a great deal of stress imparted by the continuous action of the frontalis muscle. Because of this stress, significant implant absorption is common. While theoretically thinner HA fillers such as Restylane Fine Lines and Juvéderm 18 should work well in this region, most individuals prefer CosmoDerm 1 when treating transverse forehead lines. Since the

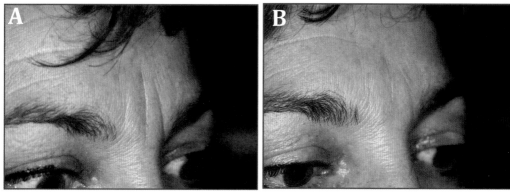

Figure 9-28. (A) Prominent central glabellar lines. (B) Two months following a Restylane injection.

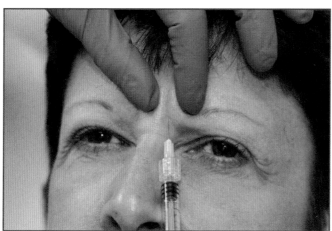

Figure 9-29. Injection of HA filler to reduce the appearance of glabellar furrows using a linear threading technique.

injection depth in this region is typically 1 mm to 2 mm, there is the potential that HA fillers will show and over-correction can occur. The implant should be placed intradermally at a depth of 1 mm to 1.5 mm with a 30-gauge needle. A serial puncture technique is utilized. Some injectors prefer to inject in the axis of the transverse forehead line while other individuals prefer administering CosmoDerm 1 perpendicular to the axis of the line. The line should be filled to the point where a white blanch is observed and an over-correction of approximately 150% should be obtained because regression will occur following treatment with CosmoDerm 1.

HA fillers may also be utilized for treating forehead lines (Figure 9-30). Topical anesthesia or a supraorbital combined with a supratrochlear nerve block (see Figure 9-16) works well in this region, similar to the treatment of vertical glabellar frown lines. The implant should be placed intradermally at a depth of 1 mm to 2 mm using a 30-gauge needle. A linear threading technique is utilized, positioning the needle parallel to the horizontal forehead line. The line should be completely filled but should never be over-corrected because this can cause postinjection ridging.

Treatment of Facial Scars

The first step in the actual treatment of acne and facial scars is to determine which lesions are likely to respond to treatment. Lesion selection is important because HA fillers afford the best results in soft, distensible lesions with gently sloping sides. The stretch test

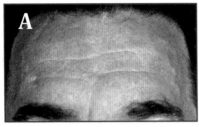
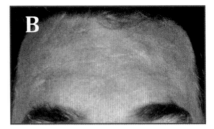

Figure 9-30. Horizontal forehead lines (A) before and (B) after treatment with CosmoDerm 1®. (Reprinted with permission of Allergan, Inc.)

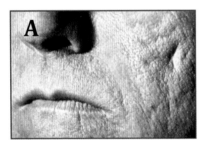
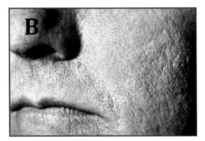

Figure 9-31. Acne scars (A) before and (B) after treatment with CosmoDerm 1®. (Reprinted with permission of Allergan, Inc.)

is useful in predicting which lesions are likely to respond: The thumb and forefinger are used to stretch the skin around a depressed scar. If stretching eliminates the defect, then correction is possible. Indurated scars do not respond as favorably initially, and several implantations may be necessary to distend the tissue. Ice pick scars do not respond well at all to filler agents.[20] In addition to the type of scar, the depth and size of the lesion must also be taken into account. Deep lesions (>5 mm) can seldom be corrected with either collagen or HA fillers.[21]

Side lighting is especially important during injection of facial scars because it highlights the depressed scars. Preinjection markings are helpful in that they help the physician to avoid injecting into the temporary valleys that have been artificially created by the collagen deposits.[9] HA fillers are typically used, although in some cases CosmoPlast may be more appropriate. The type and amount of collagen used to treat acne scars depends on the number, size, and firmness of each lesion. When using HA fillers, the material is injected at an angle of 10 degrees to 15 degrees and at a depth of 2 mm to 3 mm through a 30-gauge needle. Begin injecting within the center of the scar, raising a wheal. Withdraw the needle and then continue to inject into the portion of the scar that remains uncorrected. During implantation, a scar may become elevated to a certain level at which additional injected material spreads laterally but does not elevate the scar further. This indicates an end point for injection. Light massage following the injection may act to evenly distribute the material. A scheduled 2-week follow-up visit to enhance treatment is often necessary for improved patient satisfaction (Figure 9-31 and 9-32).

Correction of the Aging Mouth

The aging process of the mouth is associated with the development of circumoral radial grooves and a decrease in the volume of the lips themselves.[24] Soluble forms of injectable collagen such as CosmoDerm and CosmoPlast are intended for injection into the vermilion border of the lips, not within the body of the lip where they are rapidly

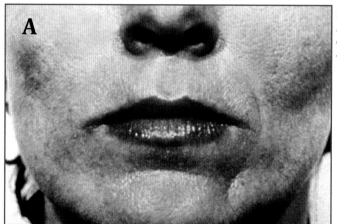

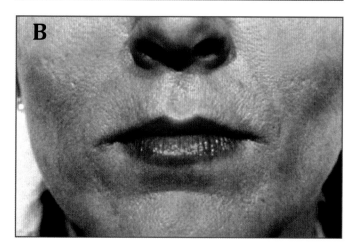

Figure 9-32. Facial scar (A) before and (B) after treatment with CosmoDerm 1® and 2®. (Reprinted with permission of Allergan, Inc.)

reabsorbed. In contrast, HA fillers may be injected just below the vermilion border into the lip itself to augment the volume of the lip. The best results are usually obtained by combining HA fillers and human collagen to simultaneously increase lip volume and define the vermilion border. Since CosmoPlast and CosmoDerm contain lidocaine, it is preferable to augment the vermilion border with these agents prior to administering HA fillers. The lidocaine that is present in the collagen fillers provides excellent supplemental anesthesia and significantly reduces the pain associated with the injection of HA fillers. For some patients with vertical "smokers lines," however, direct injection of CosmoDerm into the vertical lip lines may be necessary to maximize the treatment effect.

Augmentation of the Vermilion Border

CosmoPlast is recommended for augmenting the vermilion border since it contains lidocaine and provides excellent supplemental anesthesia for subsequent volume augmentation with a HA filler. While HA fillers may also be placed along the vermilion border, they do not contain lidocaine and will not provide pain relief for subsequent HA filler injections. It should be noted, however, that topical anesthetics and/or regional nerve blocks, including gingival injections of local anesthetic in the infraorbital (maxillary nerve) and submental regions, provide optimal patient comfort for either type of agent (see Figures 9-16 and 9-17). Unlike the serial puncture technique that is typically employed, a linear threading technique is used to deposit CosmoPlast along the vermilion border. Begin with the lower lip when augmenting the vermilion border. While injecting, grasp the lip between the thumb and forefinger. The potential space is then filled as the needle is withdrawn from the center of the lip extending to the lateral commissure. Starting at one corner, inject at a 10-degree to 15-degree angle using a 30-gauge needle. The needle is directed parallel to the mucocutaneous junction. As the needle is slowly advanced through the skin, a sudden drop in resistance signals that the needle has entered the proper plane. Once in this potential space, inject with firm and constant pressure while slowly withdrawing the needle. The material will be seen flowing from the tip of the needle within the potential space. If a spot is reached where the material will not easily advance, advance the needle slightly beyond this point and then continue to inject. Alternatively, withdraw the needle and re-enter distal to this locale. Following injection, sculpt the material by pinching the lips gently along the vermilion border. Be sure to place sufficient CosmoPlast in the lateral commissures of the lower lip because this will "lift" the corners of the mouth (Figure 9-33).[24]

The injection technique for the upper lip is similar to that of the lower lip. In the upper lip, the potential space can be entered from the corners, though some physicians prefer to enter the space centrally and inject toward the corners of the mouth. This approach will preserve the patient's natural "cupid's bow." In order to enhance the definition of the upper lip, the columns of the philtrum may be injected using either a threading or serial puncture technique. This will serve to highlight the cupid's bow and improve the 3-dimensional definition. Puragen Plus will likely replace CosmoPlast as the best agent for augmentation of the vermilion border once it becomes FDA approved since it contains both HA and lidocaine.

Lip Volume Augmentation

Once the vermilion border has been defined (and anesthetized) with CosmoPlast, the body of the lip below the vermilion border may be injected with an HA filler without additional anesthesia or supplemental topical anesthesia. Compounds that are commonly used in the United States for this purpose include Restylane, Hylaform, Captique, and Juvéderm Ultra Plus. New HA fillers will be similarly employed for this purpose as they become FDA approved. A linear threading technique is employed (Figures 9-34 to 9-36).

Frequent maintenance therapy is necessary for lip volume augmentation due to the constant stress imparted on lip tissue. Some authors feel that after repeated injections, the augmentation process in the body of the lip begins to "hold," possibly as the result of subtle fibroplasia, so that touch-ups are only necessary 2 or 3 times a year.[41]

Correction of Vertical Lip Lines

Currently, CosmoDerm 1 is recommended for treatment of vertical lip lines. The patient should purse his or her lips or whistle to accentuate these lines. The material should be injected at a 10-degree to 15-degree angle using a serial puncture technique. Direct the needle perpendicular to the line. Inject CosmoDerm 1 at a depth of 1 mm. It is okay to raise a slight wheal; however, avoid significant over-correction. Correction of up to only 100% to 150% is recommended to prevent post-treatment lumping. Use of CosmoPlast for the treatment of vertical lip lines is discouraged because it will lead to over-correction and persistent lumping within the tissue (Figure 9-37).

Post-Treatment Care

Swab the skin with alcohol or hydrogen peroxide after full correction of all treated areas has been achieved. Have the patient look at the corrected area to make certain he

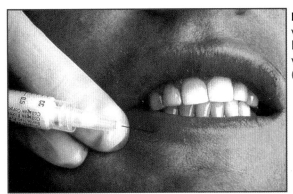

Figure 9-33. Technique of lip augmentation with CosmoPlast® injected along the vermillion border. Subsequent volume augmentation with HA fillers will provide optimal results. (Reprinted with permission of Allergan, Inc.)

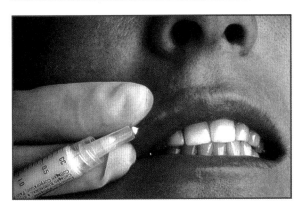

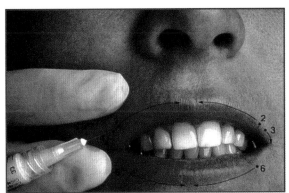

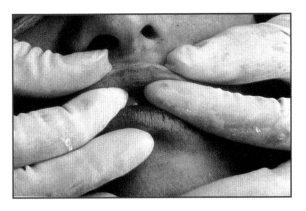

Figure 9-34. Lip volume augmentation with HA filler using a linear threading technique.

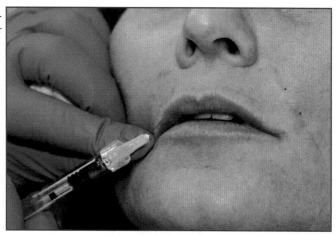

Figure 9-35. Manual massage of HA filler following lip volume augmentation.

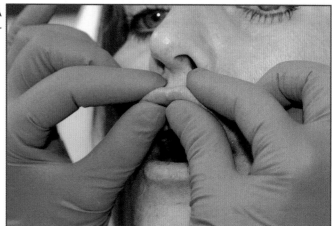

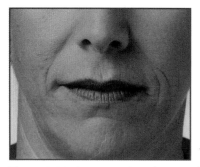 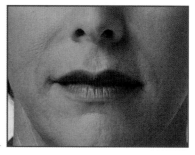

Figure 9-36. Augmentation of atropic lips with Juvéderm™. (Reprinted with permission of Allergan, Inc.)

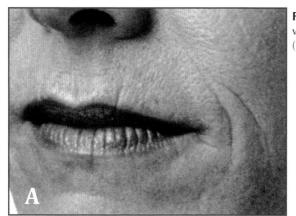

Figure 9-37. Treatment of vertical lip lines with CosmoDerm® (A) before and (B) after. (Reprinted with permission of Allergan, Inc.)

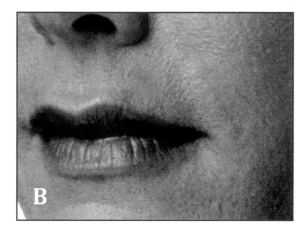

or she is satisfied with the results. Ice packs may be helpful for decreasing post-treatment discomfort and for constricting the injection sites so make-up can be applied soon after. It is acceptable for patients to cover the treated area with make-up within a few hours after injection. Patients should avoid strenuous exercise, excessive heat exposure, and alcohol consumption for the first 24 hours after treatment as these activities may cause temporary redness, swelling, or itching near the injection site. Appropriate information regarding the treatment session should be recorded in the patient's treatment record. This information should include the specific areas treated, type of material used, number and sizes of syringes used, and syringe lot numbers. Any adverse events or reactions should be noted.

Semipermanent Biodegradeable Agents

The advantage of these compounds is their increased duration of effect, which typically lasts 1 to 2 years. Their drawbacks and limitations, however, include increased expense, difficulty of use, and steeper learning curve for practitioners as well as multiple treatments and a higher incidence of severe complications, including granuloma and nodule formation. At present, 2 of these agents (Radiesse and Sculptra) are not FDA approved for cosmetic use and are, therefore, used in an off-label fashion as dermal filler agents.

Fascian™ (Fascia Biosytems, LLC, Beverly Hills, Calif) is a human tissue product (preserved fascia) and does not require FDA approval. For this reason, injection techniques will be limited to the use of Fascian, which has been available since 1999.

FASCIAN

Fascian is an injectable lyophilized, particulate human fascia lata derived from human cadavers.[42] Unlike soluble forms of injectable collagen, Fascian represents an insoluble material that is intended to stimulate collagen production within the recipient tissue. The generation of native collagen in response to the insertion of a stimulator material is known as "recollagenation."[43] Histologic studies have confirmed that small pieces of fascia lata implanted intradermally are digested as an extraneous tissue and then replaced with native collagen in time (Figure 9-38).[44]

Fascian is harvested from cadaveric tissue. Donor suitability has been determined by the donating tissue bank according to the standards of the American Association of Tissue Banks (AATB) and the US FDA. According to these criteria, donor serum must be negative by FDA-licensed tests for human immunodeficiency virus antibody (anti-HIV 1-2), Hepatitis B surface antigen (HBsAG), hepatitis B core antibody (HBcAB), hepatitis C antibody (anti HCV), human T-lymphotropic virus type I antibody (anti HTLV-1), and rapid plasma reagin (RPR) for syphilis. The risk of transmission of infectious disease is reduced further by preirradiation of the implant with 1.5 to 1.8 megarads and sterilization with ethylene oxide.[42]

The graft is particulated (ground, not pulverized) into predetermined sizes and then freeze-dried to a water content of less than 6%. It is then loaded into a 3-cc syringe and vacuum packaged for shipping and storage at room temperature.

Syringes of 5 different particle sizes (2.0 mm, 1.0 mm, 0.5 mm, 0.25 mm, and 0.1 mm) are available, each containing 80 mg of material per syringe. The larger particles are believed to be more likely to be replaced with native collagen, as compared to the smaller particle sizes. As a result, there may be less absorption and greater long-term tissue augmentation with larger particle sizes. On the other hand, the smaller particle sizes have less incidence of clogging the needle during the injection process and can be injected with smaller gauge needles. In most instances, the larger particle sizes are intended for subdermal injection, while smaller particles are intended for intradermal injection. It has been suggested that both the indications and longevity of duration of the larger particle size injectable are similar to that of autologous fat, while the indications and duration of effect of the smaller particle sizes are more closely match that of soluble forms of injectable collagen such as CosmoDerm and Zyderm. The appropriate particle size for injection is ultimately selected according to the surgeon's preference, the site and the tissue to be injected, and the degree of augmentation desired. For most instances, the 0.5-mm particle size injected with an 18- or 20-gauge needle is recommended.[43]

Allergenicity and Contraindications

Because Fascian is an allogeneic product, skin testing is not required. Although a handful of mild local reactions consisting of transient swelling have been reported, severe allergic reactions have not been reported. Like injectable collagen, Fascian is not recommended in pregnant patients and in children. Relative contraindications include use in patients with active infection at the injection site, active herpetic dermatitis, or history of a connective or autoimmune disease.[42] Because the implant contains trace amounts of polymyxin B sulfate, bacitracin, and/or gentamicin, it should be avoided in patients with a known allergy to these antibiotics.

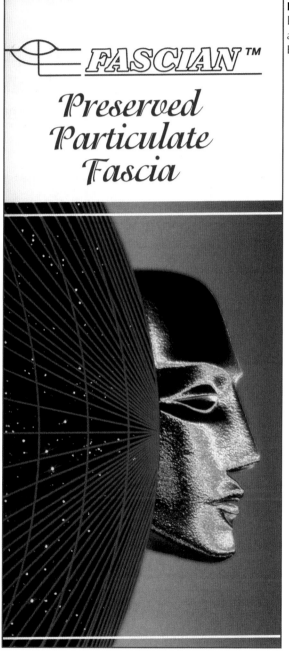

Figure 9-38. Fascian is an injectable lyophilized, particulate human fascia lata, available in 5 particle sizes. (Courtesy of Fascia Biosystems, LLC.)

Indications

Fascian may be injected intradermally, subdermally, or in deep tissue depending on the level of tissue loss; subdermal injection is preferred for larger particle sizes as more superficial injections may produce lumpiness and a persistent inflammatory response. Larger particle sizes of Fascian are most useful for upper and lower lip augmentation, treatment of deeper facial rhytides, and to fill out volume-deficient areas of the face. Smaller particle sizes of Fascian are promoted for reduction of fine lines and wrinkles. Because these smaller particles do not stimulate recollagenation, their duration of action is similar to that of injectable soluble collagen. Because superficial injection of even smaller particle sizes is more often associated with lumpiness and localized inflammation, Fascian is not recommended for the treatment of fine periocular lines.

Technique

The material is stored freeze dried so hydration of the material is necessary. Hydration is relatively simple and can be performed minutes prior to the procedure. Fascian should be hydrated by aspirating 1.0 cc of normal saline and 1 cc of 1% lidocaine with 1:100,000 dilution of epinephrine into the syringe containing the dried pellet of Fascian. A Luer-to-Luer syringe connector is next used to join a second 3-cc syringe. The material is then mixed by transferring the contents back and forth between the 2 syringes. This action conveniently stirs particles, which hydrate readily.[43] Agitating and inverting the syringe helps to progressively disperse the material from the pellet, resulting in a thick suspension of the entire contents. Adequate hydration and mixing are necessary to ensure smooth injection.

The proper needle for injection is then selected. The larger particle sizes are best injected through a 14- or 16-gauge needle, while the medium size particles pass readily through an 18- to 20-gauge needle. The smaller particle sizes easily flow through a 22- to 25-gauge needle.

The patient is readied for injection in the manner as previously described for collagen and/or HA injections. Because Fascian injections are significantly more painful than injections of soluble collagen, supplemental anesthesia using a nerve block or local infiltration of lidocaine is recommended.

Subdermal undermining or subcision with a needle tip will be necessary when depositing Fascian subdermally (Figure 9-39). When subcising, a 20-gauge or larger needle is used to enter the skin at the edge of the defect.[45] Using a single puncture site, several passes of the needle are made in a radial fashion within a subdermal plane underneath the area to be injected. Next, the bevel of the needle is used as a knife to connect the radial tunnels so that the entire area is undermined and a complete pocket is formed.[45] The material can then be easily injected into this newly created potential space (Table 9-3).

Specific Treatment Techniques

Nasolabial Folds

Fascian (0.5-mm particle size) injected through an 18-gauge needle is recommended for treatment of nasolabial folds. The implant should be deposited within a pocket created within the subdermal plane by subcision. The needle should penetrate the skin at the inferior extent of the nasolabial fold, lateral to the lip commissure. While

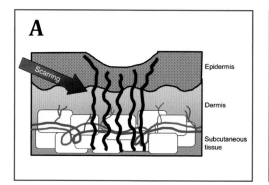
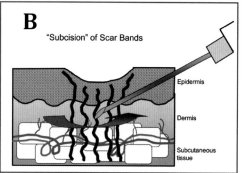
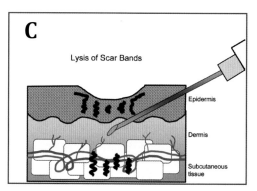
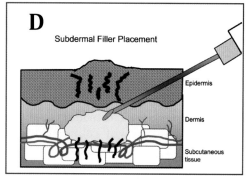

Figure 9-39. The technique of subincision. (A) A 20-gauge or larger needle is used to center the skin at the edge of the defect. (B) Using a single puncture site, several passes of the needle are made in a radial fashion within a subdermal plane underneath the area to be injected. (C) Next, with the needle down and with side-to-side sweeps of the area, the bevel of the needle is used as a knife to connect the radial tunnels so that the entire area is undermined and a complete pocket is formed. (D) The material can then be easily injected into this newly created potential space.

Table 9-3
Common Dosage Requirements for Fascian

Lip augmentation	160 mg of particles in the upper lip 80 mg of particles in the lower lip
Nasolabial fold	40 mg of particles per fold
Glabellar frown lines	80 mg of particles

maintaining inferolateral countertraction once the needle has entered the subdermal plane, the tip of the needle is advanced to the level of the ala. The bevel of the needle is swept in a side-to-side motion during advancement in order to lyse connections of the dermis to the underlying muscle and to create a pocket for the Fascian. The material is then deposited into the newly created pocket as the needle is withdrawn. Even deposition and massage will help to minimize nodule formation.[42]

Glabellar Frown Lines

Fascian (0.5-mm particle size) deposited through an 18-gauge needle is recommended for treatment of prominent glabellar lines. The needle is inserted just above the fold and then directed toward the inferior aspect of the fold in a subdermal plane. Prior to injection, horizontal undermining is important and should be performed immediately under the rhytides of concern in order to create a pocket for the material. The material is then injected evenly within the subdermal pocket as the needle is withdrawn.[44] Following injection, massage the area to spread the particles evenly.

Marionette Lines and Perioral Smile Lines

Fascian (0.1-mm to 0.5-mm particle sizes) deposited through a 20-gauge or larger needle is recommended for treatment of prominent marionette lines and perioral "smile" lines. The larger size particle mixture should be deposited in the superficial subdermal plane, while the smaller particle sizes can be injected intradermally. Smaller particle sizes can be directly injected into the dermis in a manner similar to that used for Zyplast. When treating marionette lines with larger particle sizes, the needle is inserted at the inferior aspect of the fold and then directed toward the lateral commissure. Prior to injection, horizontal undermining is necessary immediately under the rhytides of concern in order to create a pocket for the material. The material is then injected evenly within the subdermal pocket as the needle is withdrawn. Following injection, massage the area to spread the particles evenly. Perioral smile lines are treated in a similar fashion to marionette lines.

Horizontal Forehead Lines

Fascian (0.1-mm to 0.25-mm particles sizes) injected through a 20- to 22-gauge needle is used to augment horizontal forehead lines. As with soluble collagen, treatment results in this region are limited due to the stress imparted on the implant by the dynamic motion of the forehead. The horizontal line is best augmented by injecting the material intradermally using a serial puncture technique.

Lip Augmentation

An 18-gauge needle and 0.5-mm particle size Fascian are used for lip augmentation. The patient is placed in a reclining position with the neck slightly extended. The upper lip is treated first. The lip is stretched by lateral traction placed with the index finger of the hand not holding the Fascian, and a puncture wound is created just on the cutaneous side of the vermilion border at the lateral commissure. While lateral traction is maintained, the needle (bevel up) is advanced parallel to the vermilion border in a plane between the dermis and subdermal orbicularis oris muscle toward the center of the lip. The plane for injection is easily recognized as it is a natural tissue plane. Deeper injections into the muscle are not harmful, but this may cause bruising and can potentially distort the action of the muscle slightly. Superficial intradermal injections should be avoided as this may lead to nodule formation and an inflammatory response, resulting in nodularity and tenderness that can last several weeks. When advancing the needle, a slight side-to-side motion of the tip of the needle will saucerize the tissue, creating a subdermal pocket into which the Fascian is deposited. However, true subcision with the lips is unnecessary.[42-44] Prior to injecting the material, the needle should be advanced up to the hub so that the tip reaches the pillar of the philtrum where the injection is to begin. Before injection, rotate the syringe so the bevel of the needle turns 180 degrees and faces the muscle deep to the needle. The Fascian is then deposited with the bevel facing posteriorly toward the muscle. A finite amount of the Fascian suspension is then injected; the needle is then withdrawn back a small distance before the material is injected again. Small aliquots of the suspension are deposited as the needle is withdrawn. It is acceptable to reinject should areas of under-treatment exist. Each side of the upper lip is treated to the desired effect. It may be necessary to inject the cupid's bow area and the columns of the philtrum through separate stab incisions with the needle oriented vertically. When treating the pillars, advance the needle from the vermilion border cephalad toward the columella or nostrils. Fill in the pillars but do not fill in the center of the philtrum. The goal is to enhance, not flatten, the 3-dimensional contour in this area. Limited horizontal injection of cupid's bow along the vermilion will give a nice enhancement to the central area of the upper lip. Additional material may be injected submucosally within the central third of the lip in order to improve the prominence, or "pout," of the red portion of the lips. Deep injection near the muscle will prevent superficial lumping. It is important to massage the treated lip in order to obtain a uniform effect. Slight over-correction is recommended. The lower lip is treated in a similar manner following treatment of the upper lip. As a rule, the lower lip will not usually need as much volume augmentation as the upper lip (Figure 9-40).

Facial Scars and Depressions

Fascian of various particle sizes may be utilized for correcting a variety of skin depressions, including depressed scars and acne scars. Typically, a short 26-gauge needle is utilized and the material is deposited in the subdermal space using a serial puncture technique. Subcision is often necessary to lyse subcutaneous scar bands and to allow for the implant to be injected. Gentle massage of the area after implantation distributes the material evenly. Because minimal over-correction is recommended, a series of injections is required to achieve adequate augmentation (Figure 9-41).

Post-Treatment Care

Treated areas often appear over-corrected as the tissues swell. The rehydrating saline and/or local anesthetic fluids are typically reabsorbed over 1 to 3 hours. The puncture sites are cleaned with hydrogen peroxide and alcohol following injection. Firm pressure should be used to control bleeding from the puncture sights. Iced compresses are placed on the treatment area immediately and should be maintained for a minimum of 20 minutes following injection. Commonly, 3 days of antibiotics and steroids are prescribed after each treatment session.[42]

Local tenderness is minimal and limited to the day of implantation. Minimal local ecchymosis occurs sporadically. Injection site complications such as local infection, abscess, and tissue necrosis are rare, but possible. Patients may note firmness in the treated area for 1 to 2 months after injection, but visual lumpiness is rare. Local inflammatory reactions at the site of treatment are rare but may occur. Such reactions appear as excessive swelling in neighboring areas for 1 to 2 weeks after treatment and usually respond to short courses of steroids.[43] Temporary local hyperpigmentation may be anticipated in dark-skinned ethnic groups as a result of intradermal injections. This is typically transient but may persist in individuals prone to postinflammatory hyperpigmentation.

Some defects will resolve with a single treatment, but others require multiple treatments. In some cases, further maintenance injections are needed progressively less often after repeat treatments. Soft tissue augmentation with Fascian may last 3 to 4 months or longer. Larger particles demonstrate the greatest longevity of correction, whereas finer particles typically last the same length of time as injectable collagen. Some graft persistence may be evident upon repeated treatments. On average, patients should expect the need for repeat treatment at 2 to 3 months following the initial injection, then at 4 to 6 months after the second injection, and then every 6 to 7 months thereafter.

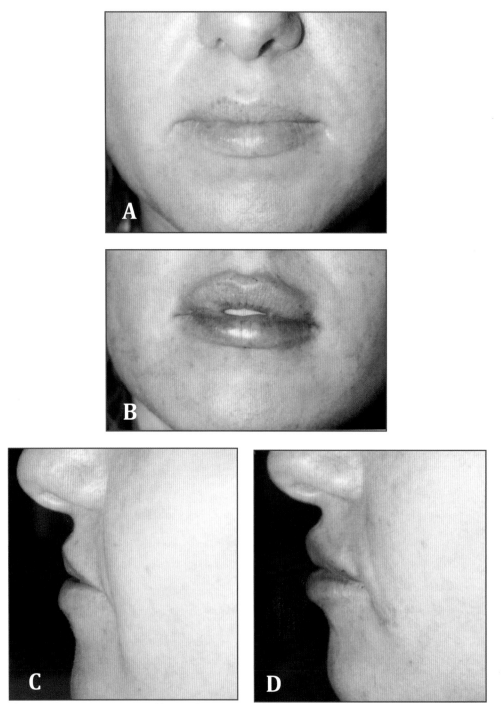

Figure 9-40. Augmentation of lips with Fascian (A) before and (B) after. Same patient, side view, (C) before and (D) after.

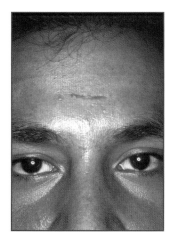 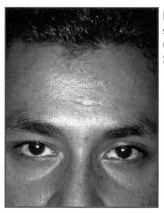

Figure 9-41. Treatment of a linear scar of the forehead with Fascian (A) before and (B) after. (Courtesy of Steven Burres.)

Calcium Hydroxyapatite Microspheres

Calcium hydroxyapatite is a major mineral component of bone and has been used for bone and craniofacial reconstruction for decades. Radiesse is a solution of 55.7% calcium hydroxyapatite microspheres (25 μm to 45 μm in diameter) that is suspended in 36.6% water for injection USP with 6.4% glycerin USP and 1.3% carboxymethylcellulose. In addition to bone augmentation, it is also used for vocal cord augmentation in cases of recurrent laryngeal nerve paresis and radiographic tissue marking. It has been found to be biocompatible and no antigenicity tests are required. Clinical trials for FDA approval for nasolabial folds are currently in place. The mechanism of action of Radiesse centers on the product being incorporated into the surrounding tissue and then being replaced through collagenesis. It is eventually broken down by hydrolytic enzymes into calcium and phosphate. Since it is relatively firm on palpation and the potential for lump and granuloma formation is significant, it is not suggested for use in lip augmentation. In addition, since it is a relatively dense material, treatment of glabellar furrows should be avoided to prevent ischemic necrosis secondary to occlusion or compression of the supraorbital and/or supratrochlear artery.

Poly-L-Lactic Acid Microspheres

PLLA is a biodegradable, synthesized corn material that has been used for decades in absorbable sutures, including polyglactin 910 and Dextran (Pharmacosmos A/S, Holbaek, Denmark) as well as craniofacial plates and screws. Following a successful launch in Europe, New-Fill was acquired by sanofi-aventis and marketed in the US in 2004 under the name Sculptra™ (Figure 9-42). Sculptra is FDA approved for the treatment of HIV facial lipodystrophy, and all other aesthetic applications are performed in an off-label fashion.

Reconstitution and Injection Technique

Sculptra/New-Fill is supplied in a dry powder form and is suspended with 5 mL of sterile water for injection (SWFI) sterile saline or lidocaine prior to administration. The vial should be allowed to stand for at least 2 hours to ensure complete hydration and should not be shaken during this period of time. The product is then agitated until a uniform translucent suspension is obtained. The reconstituted material is usable within 72 hours of reconstitution and should be agitated prior to administration. To remove the

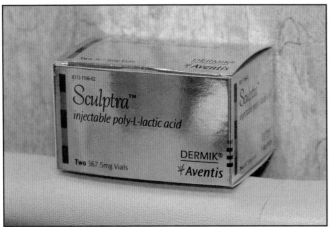

Figure 9-42. Sculptra is composed of poly-l-lactic acid (PLLA) microspheres that stimulate collagen production.

material from the vial, clean the penetrable stopper of the vial with an alcohol wipe and use a new 18-gauge, sterile needle to withdraw an appropriate amount of the suspension (typically 1 mL) into a single-use, 1-mL, sterile syringe. Do not store the reconstituted product in the syringe. Replace the 18-gauge needle with a 26-gauge, sterile needle before injecting the product into the deep dermis or subcutaneous layer. Do not inject Sculptra using needles of an internal diameter smaller than 26 gauge. Injections are reserved for the deep dermal or subcutis planes since lumps or granulomas can develop. The mechanism of action is a pure foreign body reaction that stimulates neocollagenesis, resulting in 3-dimensional volume expansion.

Anesthesia is best obtained by combining topical anesthesia with local nerve blocks as described in previous sections. To control the injection depth of Sculptra, stretch or pull the skin opposite to the direction of the injection to create a firm injection surface. A 26-gauge, sterile needle should be introduced bevel up into the skin at an angle of approximately 30 to 40 degrees until the desired skin depth is reached. A change in tissue resistance is evident when the needle traverses the dermal-subcutaneous junction. If the needle is inserted at too shallow an angle (ie, into the mid or superficial [papillary] dermis), the bevel of the needle may be visible through the skin. If Sculptra is injected too superficially, it will be evident as immediate or slightly delayed blanching in the injected area. If this occurs, the needle should be removed and the treatment area gently massaged.

When the appropriate dermal plane is reached, the needle angle should be lowered to advance the needle in that dermal plane. Prior to depositing Sculptra, a reflux maneuver should be performed to ensure that a blood vessel has not been entered. Using the threading or tunneling technique, a thin trail of Sculptra should then be deposited in the tissue plane as the needle is withdrawn. To avoid deposition in the superficial skin, deposition should be stopped before the needle bevel is visible in the skin. The treatment areas should be periodically massaged during the injection session to evenly distribute the product. It is important to note that the depressed area should never be over-corrected (overfilled) in an injection session. Typically, patients will experience some degree of edema associated with the injection procedure itself, which will give the appearance of a full correction by the end of the injection session (within about 30 minutes). The patient should be informed that the injection-related edema typically resolves in several hours to a few days, resulting in the "reappearance" of the original contour deficiency.

The volume of Sculptra should be limited to approximately 0.1 mL to 0.2 mL per each individual injection. Note that in areas such as the cheek, approximately 20 injections may be required to cover the targeted area. The volume of product injected per treatment area will vary depending on the surface area to be treated. Treatment for severe facial fat loss in patients with HIV facial lipodystrophy typically requires the injection of 1 vial of Sculptra per cheek area per injection session. Multiple injections (typically administered in a grid or cross-hatched pattern) may be required to cover the targeted area. The total number of injections and thus total volume of Sculptra injected will vary based on the surface area to be corrected, not on the depth or severity of the deficiency to be corrected.

Redness, swelling, and/or bruising may be noted in the treatment area immediately following an injection session with Sculptra. Applying an ice pack to the injected area once treatment is completed can reduce swelling. The patient should periodically massage the treatment area for several days after the injection session to promote a natural-looking correction.

Only a limited correction should be made during the first injection session with Sculptra. A typical treatment course for severe facial fat loss involves 3 to 6 injection sessions, with the sessions separated by 2 or more weeks. Full effects of the treatment course are evident within weeks to months. The patient should be re-evaluated no sooner than 2 weeks after each injection session to determine if additional correction is needed. Patients should be advised that supplemental injection sessions might be required to maintain an optimal treatment effect.

Permanent Nonbiodegradable Compounds

The ideal dermal filler agent is not essentially permanent. While a permanent agent may sound appealing at first, it is important to understand that an individual's soft tissue volume and structure change with time. One concern with administering permanent fillers is what will happen to the agent and injected area over the future potential lifespan of the patient.

POLYMETHYLMETHACRYLATE MICROSPHERES SUSPENDED IN BOVINE COLLAGEN

ArteFill consists of homogenous PMMA microspheres (20% by volume) evenly suspended in purified bovine collagen gel (80% by volume). It is a permanent, injectable soft tissue filler. All microspheres are in the range of 30 µm to 50 µm in size, are completely round, and have a smooth surface. ArteFill also contains an average 0.3% lidocaine hydrochloride. Following its injection in the lower part of the dermis, the collagen vehicle is degraded within 1 to 3 months. The microspheres subsequently become encapsulated with a fine fibrous capsule, a process that is completed within 2 to 4 months after injection. Since the PMMA microspheres are nonbiodegradable and too large to be phagocytosed or taken up by the vasculature, the resulting tissue augmentation will be long lasting.

ArteFill has been suggested for glabellar frown lines, perioral lines, lip augmentation, acne scars, etc. It is not designed for fine wrinkle lines, as it must be placed deep within the dermis. ArteFill has been recently approved by the FDA as a filling agent for the reduction of nasolabial folds (Figure 9-43). It has not been investigated for volume augmentation of the lips to date. ArteFill was found to be superior to collagen at 6 months as a filling agent for these areas.[46] Adverse events were minor in nature.

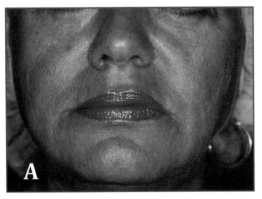
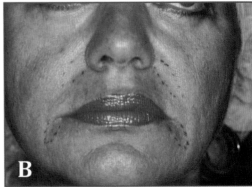

Figure 9-43. (A) Pre-ArteFill injection. (B) Areas to be injected. (C) One month post-ArteFill.

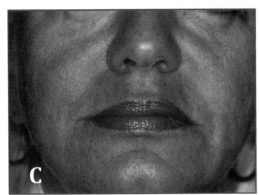

Injection Technique and Tips

The product is stored in the refrigerator and allowed to warm to room temperature over 4 hours prior to injection. Rapid warming (holding it over a heater or rubbing it between your hands) leads to clumping of the beads at one end. Experienced injectors have found that allowing the product to warm to room temperature for 8 to 15 hours actually works the best. Immediately prior to injections, the plunger on the syringe should be advanced until some of the product is seen at the needle tip. Occasionally, one cannot advance the plunger due to clogging of the needle with the product. A change in needle usually remedies the problem but also leads to a loss of some of the ArteFill. The volume to be injected depends on the depth and size of the wrinkle. A linear threading technique and/or a serial puncture technique are used to deposit the material into the tissue. Gentle massage immediately postinjection helps smooth the filler area. It is strongly advised to inform the patient that at least 2 injection sessions are required. Since the product is permanent, one does not want to over-correct the defect. It is best to aim for a partial correction; wait until the product solidifies over the next few months and then reinject to further augment the area of concern. This gradual correction of skin defects is safest and allows for a more natural, smooth, balanced result. Caution is advised because over aggressive injections may lead to irregularity or lumpiness while too superficial placement can result in permanent "beading" or "ridging."

Side Effects

As with other injectables, postinjection swelling and erythema are not unusual. Bruising occasionally occurs as well. Late side effects, including persistent redness, visibility of ArteFill through the skin, beading, and contour unevenness are infrequent and seem to be technique-related.[47] There have been recent reports of nodules or small lumps in the lips with this product, which have been a source of discomfort and annoyance to the patient.[48] In some instances, surgery was required to remove the ArteFill, an unwelcoming thought when the patient is seeking cosmetic improvement and ends up with a potentially disfiguring surgery. Some investigators are therefore concerned about its use as a soft tissue filler for lip augmentation. Careful injection into the deep dermis and avoidance of treating very thin skin will minimize the risk of beading and ridging. If significant beading or ridging occurs at the injection site, an injection of triamcinolone (2 mg/mL) may help soften and shrink the beading. Surgical excision with potential scarring is occasionally the only answer to correct the problem. Acute allergic reaction to the collagen component is rare. The reported allergic rate with ArteFill collagen is 0.78% compared with approximately 3% with Zyderm or Zyplast. It remains to be seen if the FDA will require skin testing prior to administration as this agent is currently in the final phases of FDA approval. A significant complication occasionally reported with PMMA microspheres is granuloma formation, with a reported incidence of 1 in 1000.[47] In this situation, rather than normal encapsulation of the PMMA beads occurring, a granulomatous response to the material ensues in the area of redness, inflammation, and swelling. Intralesional triamcinolone or betamethasone is required to settle the reaction.

A Return of Silicone Products?

Some individuals are taking a second look at high viscosity silicone for soft tissue filling. Two products (ADATO™ SIL 5000 [Bausch & Lomb, Rochester, NY] is 50 times thicker than water and SILIKON® 1000 [Alcon Laboratories Inc, Fort Worth, Tex] is 10 times thicker than water) are being used for lip augmentation or nasolabial folds with success. SILIKON 1000 is a highly purified injectable silicone oil. It is sterile, nonpyrogenic, clear, and colorless. SILIKON 1000 is approved by the FDA in the United States for use as a postoperative retinal tamponade during vitreoretinal surgery. SILIKON 1000 is immiscible in aqueous products, and it is relatively inert with little potential for biologic toxicity.[49] In addition, silicone has proven not to be easily contaminated with bacteria and remains sterile indefinitely.[50] Silicone is a permanent soft tissue filler. The recommended technique is to inject small amounts (0.5 cc to 1.0 cc) at a time, let it sit for a few weeks, and then reinject additional amounts depending on the desired effect. An occasional lump will occur in the injected area and reportedly responds well to a Kenalog® (Bristol-Myers Squibb, New York, NY) injection. ADATO SIL 5000 has also been useful in those AIDS patients with areas of lipodystrophy.[51]

Autologous Fat Injection

Autologous fat injections are an advanced technique for tissue augmentation. This section is intended to serve as an introduction to the technique and is not a substitute for proper training in the technique of either liposuction or successful fat implantation.

The use of autologous fat has been advocated for tissue augmentation for over a century.[52] With the introduction of tumescent liposuction in the 1970s, there has been an increased interest in utilizing the aspirated fat to augment the soft tissues of the face.[53] However, the technique of autologous fat injections has demonstrated varying success, and numerous variations in the technique of fat harvesting and fat transplantation have been described. Currently, the most popular method of soft tissue augmentation through fat transplantation is known as microlipoinjection. Microlipoinjection involves the utilization of small aspirated fat globules to augment the soft tissues of the face.[54]

INDICATIONS

Microlipoinjection is intended to correct deeper lines and furrows by injecting harvested fat into the subcutaneous tissue. Autologous fat injections are not intended for intradermal injection and are therefore contraindicated in the treatment of fine lines and wrinkles.

Clinical experience suggests that fat grafting is most successful when the fat is placed in areas already occupied with adipocytes. Sites most amenable for correction with microlipoinjection include depressed temples, hollow cheeks, deep nasolabial grooves, tear trough abnormalities, hollowed nasojugal folds, atrophic lips, and marionette lines.[54] Fat injections tend to survive best in areas with the least movement.[4]

TECHNIQUE

Most physicians feel that harvesting fat by syringe is preferable to harvesting via liposuction because of the damage to the fat cells caused by the high negative suction pressure generated with the use of high-powered aspirators. Needle size used for both harvesting and injection of fat is believed to be a strong contributor to adipocyte survival rates. The literature suggests that a transplanted fat cell survives best when either cut out and implanted as a small cylinder of tissue or aspirated and injected through a large (14-gauge or larger) bore needle (Figure 9-44).[1]

There is a great deal of individual physician variation in techniques employed for fat transplantation. However, basic steps are common to all variations of autologous fat injections: fat harvesting, fat processing, and fat injection.

Before the procedure, patients should discontinue blood thinners to reduce the risk of bruising. The first part of the procedure involves removing fat from the patient's mid to lower body area. The best sites for adipose harvest include the thighs, buttocks, medial knee, lateral flanks, and abdomen. This can be done under local anesthesia with or without an oral sedative. Anesthesia in the donor site is achieved by utilizing Klein solution (Table 9-4) (developed by Jeffrey Klein for tumescent liposuction). Adequate tumescent anesthesia will provide long-lasting anesthesia for 8 to 12 hours with effective vasoconstriction. A wide area of skin at the donor site is then prepped with povidone-iodine solution. Approximately 300 cc of Klein solution is infiltrated into the donor site. The center of the area for fat harvesting is grasped by pinching, and a puncture is made with a number 11 blade. The solution is injected through a small cannula in a radial fashion in multiple tissue planes, causing the tissue to swell and tense. The tip of the infusion cannula is constantly palpated. The fat is removed at different depths 30 minutes after injection of anesthetic with liposuction cannulas and syringes. The cannula is passed through the previously made skin puncture. The syringe of the plunger is then withdrawn and stabilized in the surgeon's hand. Alternatively, a lock can be placed on the withdrawn syringe to create negative pressure within the barrel of the syringe. With a gentle in-and-out motion, the cannula is directed in a radial, fan-shaped pattern. Normally, only 15 mL to 20 mL of material is needed. However, up to 100 cc of fat is easily harvested. Any excess fat can be frozen for up to 1 year and used for subsequent augmentation.[1]

The next step involves processing the fat. While some physicians advocate extensive washing of the harvested fat in order to reduce the inflammatory response in the recipient

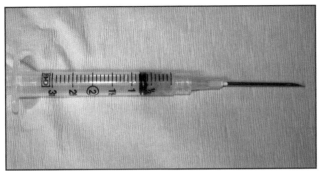

Figure 9-44. Transplanted fat cells survive best when either cut out and implanted as a small cylinder of tissue or aspirated and injected through a large (14-gauge or larger) bore needle.

Table 9-4

Klein Solution Ingredients

Ingredients	Action
1 L of normal saline	Dilatant
50 cc of lidocaine 1% plain	Anesthesia
1 mL of 1:1000 epinephrine	Vasoconstriction
10 cc of 8.4% sodium bicarbonate	Reduces the acidity and therefore discomfort of injection
0.1 cc of 10 mg/mL of Kenalog	Anti-inflammatory

bed, most prefer to allow the fat to separate in a syringe with no washing. Alternatively, the fat may be separated using gentle centrifugation.[1] Typically, the extracted liquid is left to stand vertically in 1 or more 20-cc syringes. The liquid separates into a bottom layer of serosanguineous fluid that contains mostly the Klein solution and blood, a middle layer of fat, and a thin top layer of oil. The oil and bottom fluid layers can be poured off.

For determining sites of fat injection, the patient is marked while in the seated position. A small bleb of local anesthetic is placed at each injection point of the face. For implantation, a scalpel is employed to prick the skin, and the cannula of the syringe containing fat is then inserted at this recipient site and the material injected at the level of the subcutaneous space.[1] Using a blunt-tipped liposuction cannula (which is about the size of an 18-gauge needle but without a sharp end), the surgeon injects the fat at multiple sites. The surgeon deposits fat in different planes at each planned transplant site: deep, middle, and superficial. For each cheek and lower lid, there can be as many as 50 passes, depositing fat particles that are small enough for the surrounding tissue to supply them with blood. The cannula is directed into and parallel with the surface of the skin, sliding just along the dermal-subcutaneous junction. If the defects being augmented are deep, a small tubular pocket must be created by subcision. This not only creates a tubular pocket for the placement of fat but also lyses the bound-down connective tissue. While depositing fat, pressure is applied bilaterally along the edges of the defect being filled in order to create a walled chamber for the infused fate. Molding after implantation is often necessary.[1] The site of augmentation may need a touch up with additional fat injections about 2 months after the initial treatment.

Controversy remains about the longevity of autologous fat grafts.[8,52] However, most physicians agree that successful fat transfer does provide long-lasting results. There is predictable correction of up to 25% to 50% with an average duration of about 1 year.

Swelling and bruising are fairly common at the sites of fat injection. On occasion, persistent edema, asymmetry, punctuate scarring, lumping, and bleeding may occur. Infection is rare but possible. There has been a single case of unilateral blindness reported after autologous fat transplantation presumably due to fat embolization.[55]

One of the most challenging complications of autologous fat injections is a hard lumpiness in the superficial area of the lower lid when fat is injected to correct a tear trough deformity. Because the skin in this region is very thin, it is also unforgiving. A lower strength steroid injection in the area may sometimes soften firm lumps should they occur. If not, the judicious injection of additional fat around the lump may serve to even out the area. It is far better to avoid this complication all together by keeping injections in the lower lid deep and to aim for under-correction in this region.

POSTOPERATIVE CARE

Following fat implantation, edema of the recipient tissue is common, especially within the lips and under the eyes. The patient is usually placed on a 10-day course of antibiotics. Cold compresses and elevation of the head for a minimum of 2 days aids in minimizing swelling. The most common adverse result seen with fat injection is an over- or under-correction.

> **Please see the Dermal Filler Agent Treatments videos on the accompanying DVD.**

References

1. Klein AW. Skin filling: collagen and other injectables of the skin. *Dermatol Clin.* 2001;19(3):ix, 491-508.
2. Carruthers J, Carruthers A. A prospective, randomized, parallel group study analyzing the effect of BTX-A (Botox) and nonanimal sourced HA (NASHA, Restylane) in combination compared with NASHA (Restylane) alone in severe glabellar rhytides in adult female subjects: treatment of severe glabellar rhytides with a hyaluronic acid derivative compared with the derivative and BTX-A. *Dermatol Surg.* 2003;29(8):802-809.
3. Gilcrest BA. *Skin and the Aging Process.* Boca Raton, Fla: CRC Press; 1984.
4. Carruthers JD, Carruthers A. Facial sculpting and tissue augmentation. *Dermatol Surg.* 2005;31(11 Pt 2):1604-1612.
5. De Silva LW. Erasing the years: an overview of dermal fillers. *Adv Nurse Pract.* 2006;14(2):31-33.
6. Gottlieb SK. Soft tissue augmentation: the search for implantation materials and techniques. *Clin Dermatol.* 1987;5(4):128-134.
7. Hotta T. Dermal fillers: the next generation. *Plast Surg Nurs.* 2004;24(1):14-19.
8. Kanchwala SK, Holloway L, Bucky LP. Reliable soft tissue augmentation: a clinical comparison of injectable soft-tissue fillers for facial-volume augmentation. *Ann Plast Surg.* 2005;55(1):30-35; discussion 5.
9. Narins RS, Bowman PH. Injectable skin fillers. *Clin Plast Surg.* 2005;32(2):151-162.

10. Ozgentas HE, Pindur A, Spira M, et al. A comparison of soft-tissue substitutes. *Ann Plast Surg.* 1994;33(2):171-177.

11. Wise JB, Greco T. Injectable treatments for the aging face. *Facial Plast Surg.* 2006;22(2):140-146.

12. Biesman B. Soft tissue augmentation using Restylane. *Facial Plast Surg.* 2004;20(2):171-177; discussion 8-9.

13. Duranti F, Salti G, Bovani B, et al. Injectable hyaluronic acid gel for soft tissue augmentation: a clinical and histological study. *Dermatol Surg.* 1998;24(12):1317-1325.

14. Flageul G, Halimi L. [Injectable collagen: an evaluation after 10 years' use as a complement of plastic surgery.] *Ann Chir Plast Esthet.* 1994;39(6):765-771.

15. Lindqvist C, Tveten S, Bondevik BE, Fagrell D. A randomized, evaluator-blind, multicenter comparison of the efficacy and tolerability of Perlane versus Zyplast in the correction of nasolabial folds. *Plast Reconstr Surg.* 2005;115(1):282-289.

16. Bauman L. CosmoDerm/CosmoPlast (human bioengineered collagen) for the aging face. *Facial Plast Surg.* 2004;20(2):125-128.

17. Burgess LP, Goode RL. Injectable collagen. *Facial Plast Surg.* 1992;8(3):176-182.

18. Karam P, Kibbi AG. Collagen injections. *Int J Dermatol.* 1992;31(7):467-470.

19. Keefe J, Wauk L, Chu S, DeLustro F. Clinical use of injectable bovine collagen: a decade of experience. *Clin Mater.* 1992;9(3-4):155-162.

20. Matti BA, Nicolle FV. Clinical use of Zyplast in correction of age- and disease-related contour deficiencies of the face. *Aesthetic Plast Surg.* 1990;14(3):227-234.

21. Elson ML. Clinical assessment of Zyplast implant: a year of experience for soft tissue contour correction. *J Am Acad Dermatol.* 1988;18(4 Pt 1):707-713.

22. Stegman SJ, Chu S, Bensch K, Armstrong R. A light and electron microscopic evaluation of Zyderm collagen and Zyplast implants in aging human facial skin: a pilot study. *Arch Dermatol.* 1987;123(12):1644-1649.

23. Clark DP, Hanke CW, Swanson NA. Dermal implants: safety of products injected for soft tissue augmentation. *J Am Acad Dermatol.* 1989;21(5 Pt 1):992-998.

24. Kligman AM, Armstrong RC. Histologic response to intradermal Zyderm and Zyplast (glutaraldehyde cross-linked) collagen in humans. *J Dermatol Surg Oncol.* 1986;12(4):351-357.

25. Belange G, Elbaz JS. [The role of an immunologic survey prior to using collagen implants. Theoretical aspects and practical methods.] *Ann Chir Plast Esthet.* 1989;34(1):69-72.

26. Elson ML. The role of skin testing in the use of collagen injectable materials. *J Dermatol Surg Oncol.* 1989;15:301-303.

27. Klein AW. In favor of double testing. *J Dermatol Surg Oncol.* 1989;15:263.

28. Approval letter released by the FDA regarding CosmoDerm and CosmoPlast to INAMED medical corporation. v. 2003.

29. Lowe NJ, Maxwell CA, Lowe P, et al. Hyaluronic acid skin fillers: adverse reactions and skin testing. *J Am Acad Dermatol.* 2001;45(6):930-933.

30. Coleman SR. Cross-linked hyaluronic acid fillers. *Plast Reconstr Surg.* 2006;117(2):661-665.

31. Brown LH, Frank PJ. What's new in fillers? *J Drugs Dermatol.* 2003;2(3):250-253.

32. Niamtu J 3rd. The use of Restylane in cosmetic facial surgery. *J Oral Maxillofac Surg.* 2006;64(2):317-325.

33. Lowe NJ, Maxwell CA, Patnaik R. Adverse reactions to dermal fillers: review. *Dermatol Surg.* 2005;31(11 Pt 2):1616-1625.

34. Monheit GD. Hylaform: a new hyaluronic acid filler. *Facial Plast Surg.* 2004;20(2):153-155.

35. Raulin C, Greve B, Hartschuh W, Soegding K. Exudative granulomatous reaction to hyaluronic acid (Hylaform). *Contact Dermatitis.* 2000;43(3):178-179.

36. Bergeret-Galley C, Latouche X, Illouz YG. The value of a new filler material in corrective and cosmetic surgery: DermaLive and DermaDeep. *Aesthetic Plast Surg.* 2001;25(4):249-255.

37. Andre P, Lowe NJ, Parc A, et al. Adverse reactions to dermal fillers: a review of European experiences. *J Cosmet Laser Ther.* 2005;7(3-4):171-176.

38. Schanz S, Schippert W, Ulmer A, et al. Arterial embolization caused by injection of hyaluronic acid (Restylane). *Br J Dermatol.* 2002;146(5):928-929.

39. Hanke CW, Higley HR, Jolivette DM, et al. Abscess formation and local necrosis after treatment with Zyderm or Zyplast collagen implant. *J Am Acad Dermatol.* 1991;25(2 Pt 1):319-326.

40. Smith KC, Melnychuk M. Five percent lidocaine cream applied simultaneously to the skin and mucosa of the lips creates excellent anesthesia for filler injections. *Dermatol Surg.* 2005;31(11 Pt 2):1635-1637.

41. Klein AW. In search of the perfect lip: 2005. *Dermatol Surg.* 2005;31(11 Pt 2):1599-1603.

42. Burres S. Fascian. *Facial Plast Surg.* 2004;20(2):149-152.

43. Burres S. Soft-tissue augmentation with Fascian. *Clin Plast Surg.* 2001;28(1):101-110.

44. Shore JW. Injectable lyophilized particulate human fascia lata (Fascian) for lip, perioral, and glabellar enhancement. *Ophthal Plast Reconstr Surg.* 2000;16(1):23-27.

45. Orentrich DS, Orentrich N. Subcutaneous incisionless (subcision) surgery for the correction of depressed scars and wrinkles. *Dermatol Surg.* 1995;21:543-549.

46. Cohen S. Artecoll. Panel on soft Tissue Fillers. Presented at: Advances in Aesthetic Facial and Reconstructive Plastic Surgery; 2003; Snowbird, Utah.

47. Lemperle G, Hazan-Gauthier N, Lemperle N. PMMA microspheres (Artecoll) for long term correction of wrinkles: refinements and statistical results. *Aesthetic Plast Surg.* 1998;22:356-365.

48. Blanchard M. Filler material may cause nodules, lumps in lips. *Cosmetic Surgery Times.*

49. Pollack SV. Silicone, fibrel, and collagen implantation for facial lines and wrinkles. *J Dermatol Surg Oncol.* 1990;16(10):957-961.

50. Webster RC, Gaunt JM, Hamden US, et al. Injectable silicone for facial soft tissue augmentation. *Arch Otolaryngol Head Neck Surg.* 1986;112:290-296.

51. Jones D. HIV facial lipoatrophy: causes and treatment options. *Dermatol Surg.* 2005;31(11 Pt 2):1519-1529; discussion 29.

52. Sclafani AP, Romo T 3rd. Collagen, human collagen, and fat: the search for a three-dimensional soft tissue filler. *Facial Plast Surg.* 2001;17(1):79-85.

53. Phillips PK, Pariser DM, Pariser RJ. Cosmetic procedures we all perform. *Cutis.* 1994;53(4):187-191.

54. Pinski KS, Coleman WP. Microlipoinjection and autologous collagen. Dermatol Clin. 1995;13(2):339-351.

55. Teimourian B. Blindness following fat injections (Letter). *Plast Reconstr Surg.* 1988;82:361.

Marketing Botulinum Toxin and Dermal Filler Agents to Build Your Practice

William J. Lipham, MD, FACS

In addition to acquiring the skills required to effectively evaluate and treat patients with botulinum toxin and dermal filler agents, it is also important to learn how these services can be marketed and integrated into your medical practice. This chapter will focus on both internal and external marketing techniques in order to allow you to increase patient awareness and interest in pursuing these elective treatments. While marketing has traditionally been frowned upon in the medical arena, aesthetic and cosmetic procedures are publicly perceived as services that are inherently elective in nature. As such, it is necessary for the practitioner to provide individuals with information so that they can make an informed decision about pursuing these treatment options. This chapter will focus on both internal and external marketing techniques that will allow practitioners to recruit and maintain a new pool of patients that are interested in these minimally invasive facial rejuvenation techniques.

Overall Marketing Strategy

Whether you are a dermatologist, facial plastic surgeon, oculoplastic surgeon, or general medical practitioner, it is important to understand how you can integrate botulinum toxin treatments for cosmetic and functional purposes as well as dermal filler agents into your current medical practice. For some individuals, such as dermatologists or facial plastic surgeons who already provide a variety of cosmetic and aesthetic procedures, integrating these procedures into your practice will be relatively easy. The majority of patients who are interested in these services will actively investigate and look to these types of physicians since they are perceived by the lay public as the primary group of specialists who perform these procedures. In contrast, ophthalmic plastic and reconstructive surgeons as well as otorhinolaryngologists and general practitioners will need to educate and inform the general public that they perform these procedures as well, and that they are capably trained to evaluate and treat this patient population.

Currently, there are 3 broad groups of marketing that can be used to promote cosmetic or aesthetic services into a medical practice. These include external marketing, Web-based marketing, and internal marketing. When most people think of marketing products or services, they think of external marketing, which includes television, radio, and print advertising. While these avenues may bring in a new group of patients to your practice, the cost/benefit analysis will demonstrate that a greater amount of money has to be spent to recruit a new patient utilizing these media formats. At present, many individuals, especially cosmetic and aesthetic services consumers, actively investigate the options that are available to them in the local community through the Internet. Establishing a Web page for your practice is a very cost-effective means to promote not only botulinum toxin and dermal filler agents but also your entire array of services. The most cost-effective means to introduce new patients to these treatments is to utilize internal marketing such as informational brochures, data mining, and waiting room posters and displays to promote these products to your current customer base. Research has shown that this is the most cost-effective means of marketing since you have already established a positive relationship with the individuals in your practice who may be interested in pursuing additional aesthetic treatments. Since you have an established level of trust as well as a relationship with these individuals, it is relatively easy to introduce them to the concept that they can benefit from your new array of services.

External Marketing

Unless you are starting a new practice from scratch, external marketing is a relatively expensive way to capture a new target market for a variety of goods and services. If you already have an established medical practice, your money will be better spent developing a Web page to introduce your patients to your new aesthetic procedures as well as internal marketing to drive them to your business Web site. External marketing is primarily composed of television, radio, and print advertising. For most individuals pursuing elective cosmetic or aesthetic surgical procedures, television advertising is an extremely expensive endeavor and unless pursued with a large investment, generally yields poor results in terms of generating new patient referrals. Consumers have become quite savvy at analyzing video content and expect high-level video content in order to provoke interest in pursuing a follow-up or lead. Most practitioners would find that it is quite expensive to pursue television production as a cost-effective media to promote external referrals. In general, it is best to have large corporations such as Allergan promote BOTOX cosmetic on television through tastefully placed advertisements, which will direct consumers to the BOTOX cosmetic Web site, which will then link them to your practice.

In contrast to television advertising, radio and print advertising can be significantly more cost effective and generate a reasonable rate of return with respect to new patient visits to your office. While radio advertisement slots are relatively inexpensive, most individuals considering cosmetic or aesthetic surgical procedures require more information than a radio advertisement can provide. Radio advertisements are often a useful adjunct to plant a practice name in the mind of a prospective individual who will then learn more about that person's practice through print advertising and/or Web-based information.

Print advertising is probably the most cost-effective means to promote botulinum toxin injections and dermal filler agents to the general public. News print media can be relatively expensive and targets a broad section of society that may not be interested in aesthetic procedures. In contrast, local community magazines that are aimed at a more upscale market will, in general, yield the best results. These publications have a target audience for individuals who make a certain level of income and are more likely to pursue cosmetic and aesthetic surgical procedures. These publications typically promote cosmetic or

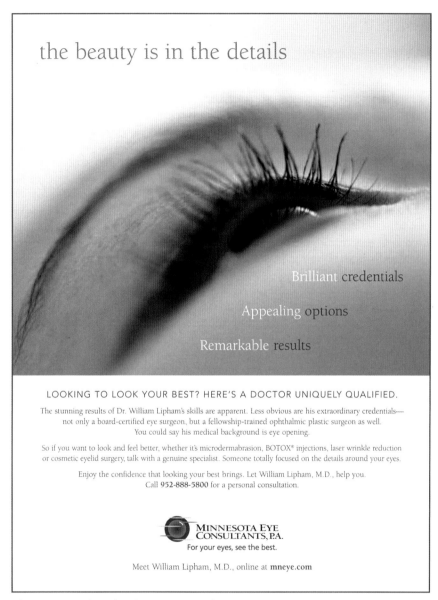

Figure 10-1. Print advertisement example.

aesthetic services 1 to 2 times per year and since they are essentially "coffee table" magazines, they allow the subscriber to review the publication and advertisement over time, which is more likely to generate a positive response and a visit to your office. In order to promote your services to Web-savvy consumers, it is imperative to include not only your phone number but also your Web address in these advertisements. Many individuals may pursue additional information about you and your practice online. In general, it is best to provide an eye-catching graphic with a mild-to-moderate amount of information rather than to overwhelm a consumer with a significant amount of detail regarding the evaluation and treatment of his or her condition. An example of a print advertisement that I have recently placed for my own services reinforces this concept (Figure 10-1).

WEB-BASED CONTENT

While older baby boomers dominate the market for functional procedures, younger baby boomers (ages 40 to 50) and Gen-X individuals (ages 30 to 40) interested in cosmetic botulinum toxin and dermal filler agents are quite Web savvy. As such, it is imperative that your practice promote these services through a Web site to provide individuals with information that they can pursue on a leisurely basis. In my opinion, both internal and external marketing are mechanisms by which you can drive individuals of the 30-to-50 year demographic toward your Web content, which can provide them with a more personalized representation of your treatment views and philosophies. Most individuals will not attempt to find local practitioners through a Web search alone, but this is changing. For example, BOTOX cosmetic has effectively established themselves in this arena by directing patients to www.botoxcosmetic.com. If an individual searches for local physicians providing BOTOX injections, they will likely be directed toward the Allergan Web site, which lists practitioners who are recommended in their geographic region.

As such, it would behoove any practitioner who is interested in performing these services to make sure that he or she is listed on the parent Web page. To do so, it may be necessary to undergo additional certification or training through a BOTOX cosmetic-approved practitioner in order to be listed on his or her Web page. It is also reasonable to consider creating your own Web page that describes the broad array of cosmetic and facial rejuvenation services that you provide. Once a consumer is logged into your Web page, he or she can peruse the content and make an informed decision about whether or not he or she would like to contact you personally. Typically, if an individual feels comfortable enough to contact you initially regarding an aesthetic procedure, he or she will very likely continue to follow up with you for repeat treatments unless there is an adverse outcome.

INTERNAL MARKETING

By far the most cost-effective means of marketing these services to your patients is through an internal approach. Internal marketing consists of in-office brochures and displays, seminars, or internal mailings to patients who are currently under your care. Since these individuals already have a positive relationship with you with respect to the other services that you provide, these approaches will be the most cost efficient. In addition, there is also a level of trust that you have established with these individuals that makes them particularly inclined to select you to perform these types of elective procedures. I feel that an who is performing BOTOX and/or dermal filler injections should have literature regarding these procedures in the form of pamphlets available at his or her offices. I frequently encounter patients in my practice who state that they became interested in pursuing these treatment options simply because they read a brochure that describes the advantages of pursuing these procedures in our office. Whenever I meet a new BOTOX cosmetic or dermal filler patient, I always make it a point to ask him or her, "How did you learn about my practice?" This is important information that will provide you with feedback as to what aspect of your marketing campaign is working most efficiently. I actually keep a running tabulation of my referral sources so I can determine which approaches are working best.

Chart-based data mining provides a more direct approach to reach a particular demographic that may be interested in these types of procedures. In our office, we data mine patients based on the types of procedures they have previously had performed as well as their age. For example, a reasonable data mine of our current patient records would include male and female individuals from the age of 35 to 50 who are interested in improving their vision with refractive surgery. Our practice sends out quarterly informational brochures to these individuals regarding the cosmetic and aesthetic services that I provide.

Data mining for these types of patients can be accomplished by scanning your database for individuals who meet favorable demographics for botulinum toxin and dermal filler agents. Typically these individuals are 35 to 50 years of age and have disposable income. Since our practice is largely refractive surgical in nature, a review of individuals who have pursued refractive surgical procedures within the age parameters previously stated are reasonable candidates to receive an informational brochure regarding these new services. Whether you are a dermatologist, facial plastic surgeon, oculoplastic surgeon, or general practitioner, you should be able to similarly mine your patient data to find a demographic that would be interested in pursuing noninvasive aesthetic procedures.

Summary

While it may serve our egos as practitioners to see our "name in lights" with external marketing, a careful review of the situation would reveal that it is more cost effective to internally market to your own loyal patient database. These direct-marketing approaches include office brochures, informational seminars, and data mining to directly mail informational content to your patients that will also direct them to a Web site that you have developed that describes your services in greater detail. The cost associated with this marketing approach includes Web page development as well as purchasing or creating in-office brochures to promote your new line of services. An additional expenditure may include print advertisement in the form of local, upscale, monthly "coffee table" magazines that serve to direct a new line of business toward your Web-based marketing effort. By implementing all of these techniques into your practice, you should be able to increase your patient base for a variety of elective procedures.

Index